Seven Blessed Habits to
RADICAL
WELLNESS

*How to Tackle the Threats to
your Health and Happiness*

Libni A. Cerdenio

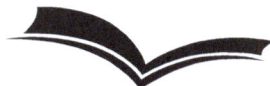

TEACH Services, Inc.
P U B L I S H I N G
www.TEACHServices.com ● (800) 367-1844

Copyright © 2021 Libni A. Cerdenio
Copyright © 2021 TEACH Services, Inc.
ISBN-13: 978-1-4796-1264-2 (Paperback)
ISBN-13: 978-1-4796-1265-9 (ePub)
Library of Congress Control Number: 2021901597

Published by

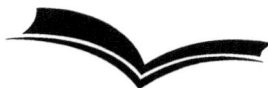

TEACH Services, Inc.
PUBLISHING
www.TEACHServices.com • (800) 367-1844

Dedication

To my wife Beth—
God's godly, loving and
beautiful gift to me
as a helpmate
for the journey.

Table of Contents

Foreword

L ibni A. Cerdenio is an authority on the topic he finely dissected which in general was the coupling of achieving excellent physical with spiritual health—being educated both in theology and as a nurse. He is a gifted writer and has it all to publish a remarkable book which I know many would be interested to read.

I like the format as it is reader friendly. The author is able to expound on his radical wellness advocacy clearly from his own perspective based on his wealth of experience, education, mentorship, conferences attended, and knowledge gleaned from media, journals, and books.

I like the way the health emphasis glides into the spiritual connection in each chapter. The messages are profound. I had to read each line slowly and a few times over in some parts to clearly get the message. Both the historical and biblical quotes and references in the book are most apt. The explanations are very well understood.

I especially love the personal experiences the author shared—especially the strong examples of answered prayers. I really love that. Those personal stories make the chapters more interesting to read.

I think the author did well on the medical science. He was able to clearly elucidate on what needed to be. Not lengthy but to the point.

I thank the author for giving me the opportunity to read this well-written, well-researched book with a most relevant message for our times. The strong spiritual overtone at the end wraps it all up positively:

"My dear friends, if we accept Jesus Christ into our lives, we receive God's gift of radical wellness. For He "came that … [we] may have life and have it abundantly" (John 10:10, ESV)."

May Ann Segovia Lao, MD.

Preface

In the early 1970s, I sat in a Philosophy of Health class taught by the late Dr. Mervyn G. Hardinge, founding dean of the then School of Health (now School of Public Health) of Loma Linda University, at the then Seventh-day Adventist Theological Seminary, Far East—now Adventist International Institute of Advanced Studies (AIIAS).

During one class session, Dr. Hardinge challenged his students to integrate the teaching of doctrine with the principles of health in the Bible. That assignment was at the back of my mind through the years of my development journalism work editing the *Health & Home* magazine in the Philippines and during my career in healthcare in the United States of America.

When I began to get involved in presenting public lectures on health, I formulated the GARDENS© integrative model of health promotion and education. It is an acronym representing the seven elements of the theocentric framework of the health and wellness ministry and advocacy which my wife Elizabeth and I have embraced in our retirement. We view this ministry and advocacy as an extension of our professional roles as registered nurses and a fulfillment of our civic duty as citizens of the world.

Instead of beginning with disease, drugs or anatomy and physiology, we believe that health promotion and education should start, continue and end with God and what He has provided for our health and happiness as revealed in the Bible and affirmed by scientific research.

We believe that radical wellness is a gift that we have to accept from God—the Giver of all good gifts. That precious gift is a blessing that comes with believing in and trusting God the Father and Jesus Christ. It is a benefit from accepting His Word, the Bible, as truth and the standard of life.

The Bible says, "Trust in the LORD with all your heart, and do not lean on your own understanding. In all your ways acknowledge him, and he will make straight your paths" (Prov. 3:5-6, ESV).

Our vision for *Seven Blessed Habits to Radical Wellness* is to inform, inspire and encourage our readers to know the basis of how to live life to its fullest.

I would like to add that this approach to health affirms true principles, the understanding and practice of which helps one avoid the traps of this generation's vigorous quest for health and wellness.

My motivation for writing this book is based on the following core values:

- *God*—I believe in a benevolent God who created the universe and continues to sustain life on this planet.
- *Purpose*—I believe that God has a design and purpose for human life and for everyone who is born in the world.
- *Knowledge*—I believe God has revealed His design and purpose in nature and in His special revelation, the Bible.
- *Community*—I believe that helping one another enhances our quality of life.

The illness-wellness continuum is a paradigm that shows not only where people may be in their state of health, but also where the different health professionals factor and practice in.

Medical practitioners range from preventive to therapeutic and crisis medicine specialists. *Seven Blessed Habits to Radical Wellness* teaches principles of health and wellness and may well be categorized with preventive intervention. It may be classified as "nomothetic medicine." The word "nomothetic" comes from two Greek words, *nomos* (laws or principles) and *thetes* (teacher). I would like to be considered as a teacher of the principles and laws of radical health and wellness.

My models and mentors in radical wellness are the following: my Lord and Savior Jesus Christ, who did a wholistic ministry during His sojourn on planet earth some 2,000 years ago; Walter Comm, my first teacher on health in college; Lester Lonergan, medical missionary in the Philippines during my college years; Hedrick Edwards, my professor and dean emeritus of the School of Health at Adventist University of the Philippines; Mervyn Hardinge, my seminary professor in Philosophy of Health who inspired me to formulate the GARDENS© integrated model of health promotion and education; Hans Diehl, whose seminars on nutrition and health I attended at the Loma Linda University Church.

I would like to thank the memory of the late James Joiner and his family for underwriting my studies in the seminary without which I wouldn't have had the experience of sitting under learned and spiritual mentors. I would especially like to honor the memory of the late Elsa Lonergan who hosted many informal teaching moments in her home, complete with healthful avocado-and-jackfruit-laden sandwiches. Above all, I would like to honor and praise God for leading me into this radical wellness ministry.

Libni A. Cerdenio
May 11, 2020
Loma Linda, California

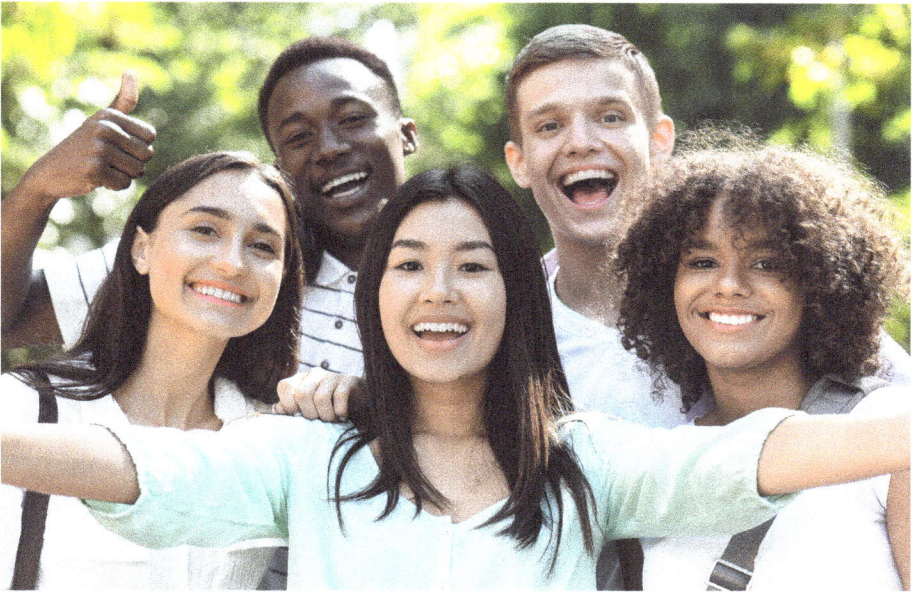

Introduction

In 1543, Nicolaus Copernicus' book, *De revolutionibus orbium coelestium libri VI*[1] (*Six Books Concerning the Revolutions of the Heavenly Orbs*), came off the press. It proposed the heliocentric (sun-centered) versus the geocentric (earth-centered) view of cosmology that was prevalent in his time. Copernicus' pioneering studies paved the way for the basic human understanding of the solar system. Today, children studying elementary astronomy know that the earth revolves around the sun, and not otherwise.

When Copernicus promulgated the heliocentric view, he added nothing to the reality of the sun and the planets revolving around it; he just provided a proper way of looking at the solar system. In a similar way, *Seven Blessed Habits to Radical Wellness* does not change the reality of what constitutes health, but it offers a better way of understanding what it really is.

Traditionally, the pursuit of health and wellness has been dominated by a man-centered world view. Policies and procedures are made and practices done with man at the center of the healthcare system.

---

[1] Nicolaus Copernicus, 1543, https://1ref.us/1ed (accessed November 2, 2020).

Our health status does not depend on our own effort and initiative but on what God has done for and given to us. All the basic support systems for us to live and thrive—air, water, sunshine, food—were provided by God at Creation. Even the beneficial physiological effects that come when we exercise, eat plant-based foods and do other health-enhancing practices are built in our bodies which are "fearfully *and* wonderfully made" by God (Ps. 139:14). Therefore, health and wellness are essentially a reality—a gift—that we need to accept and receive from God who is the Source, Sustainer and Healer of our life, health and happiness. It is a truth to be lived out because of His amazing grace and by the power of the love of Jesus Christ who "came that ... [we] may have life and have it abundantly" (John 10:10, ESV). This is what *Seven Blessed Habits to Radical Wellness* is all about.

Radical wellness is ensconced in what the apostle Paul exclaimed as God's "indescribable gift" to us—Jesus Christ our Savior and Lord (2 Cor. 9:15, NIV). Because of His great love for us, God has made us alive together with Him, not because of our works but by His grace, lest anyone should boast (Eph. 2:1–9). Consequently, we ought to live as a new person, walking in wisdom and living our lives as an expression of thanksgiving and gratitude for the exceedingly abundant life He has gifted us in Jesus Christ (Eph. 4:17–6:20). We can live thus because the love of Christ constrains us (2 Cor. 5:14). He strengthens us to do all things for His glory and for our blessing (Phil. 4:13).

God gives us good gifts because He loves us. Consider this:

The power of God is manifested in the beating of the heart, in the action of the lungs, and in the living currents that circulate through the thousand different channels of the body. We are indebted to Him for every moment of existence, and for all the comforts of life. The powers and abilities that elevate man above the lower creation, are the endowment of the Creator. He loads us with His benefits. We are indebted to Him for the food we eat, the water we drink, the clothes we wear, the air we breathe. Without His special providence, the air would be filled with pestilence and poison. He is a bountiful benefactor and preserver. The sun which shines upon the earth, and glorifies all nature, the weird solemn radiance of the moon, the glories of the firmament, spangled with brilliant stars, the showers that refresh the land, and cause vegetation to flourish, the precious things of nature in all their varied richness, the lofty trees, the shrubs and plants, the waving grain, the blue sky, the green earth, the changes of day and night, the renewing seasons, all speak to man of his Creator's love. He has linked us to Himself by all these tokens in heaven and in earth.[2]

In the beginning, God gave man the gift of good health. As Dr. Mervyn Hardinge, founding dean of the School of Public Health at Loma Linda University said: "Health came first; disease is an interloper. It came when sin entered the world, when man began to violate moral and spiritual law."[3]

In the Gift of His Son Jesus Christ, God has offered to give back the gift that the human race lost when Adam and Eve sinned.

Propositions on what constitutes a healthy life have been changing over time; new models of teaching and promoting health and wellness have been designed and promulgated; new standards of practice have been established.

Every model of health and wellness has its own good points, but I suggest that approaching the subject of health from a humanistic point of view would be like the proverbial blind men who got to feel an elephant for the first time. To the man who got its belly, the elephant was like a wall; to the one who got its ear, the elephant was like a fan; and to the one who got its leg, the elephant was like a tree.[4]

Seven Blessed Habits to Radical Wellness proposes that the best and beneficial way to real health is to learn the principles by which human beings were created and designed by God to live and function.

In *The Sound of Music*, there is an instance of profound wisdom when Governess Maria, in teaching the von Trapp children how to sing says, "When we read, we begin with A, B, C. When we sing, we begin with Do, Re, Mi ...."[5] It would be wise to follow that process in trying to discover radical wellness.

The Bible says that God created man with a three-dimensional personality—body, mind and spirit. This truth is clearly pronounced in the summary of Jesus Christ, the Model of man's growth and development: "And Jesus increased in wisdom and in stature and in favor with God and man" (Luke 2:52, ESV). Man is not only flesh and blood. He is a

[2]Ellen G. White, *Sons and Daughters of God* (Hagerstown, MD: Review and Herald, 1983), p. 17.
[3]M. Hardinge, *A Philosophy of Health* (Loma Linda, CA: School of Health, Loma Linda University, 1980), p. 1.
[4]J. Saxe, *The poems of John Godfrey Saxe* (Boston, MA: Houghton, Mifflin and Company, 1881), pp. 251–261.
[5]Robert Wise, producer and director, *The Sound of Music*, 20th Century Fox, 1965.

body, mind and spirit all in one. Total health then is defined by what God originally intended for man to be—physically, mentally, socially and spiritually.

John B. Wong attests to this proposition when he wrote his book *Christian Wholism: Theological and Ethical Implications in the Postmodern World* in the context of "our spiritual, intellectual, physical, ethical, psychological, and other domains of our multidimensional personhood."[6]

Ellen G. White began promoting what she called "health reform" at the turn of the twentieth century. Beginning in 1863, she wrote volumes on the need, nature and purpose of healthful living. In summing up her views, Angel Manuel Rodriguez, former director of the Biblical Research Institute of the General Conference of Seventh-day Adventists wrote that "Humans do not have body, mind and soul, but they are body mind, and soul."[7] He quotes her belief in the interconnectedness of these dimensions of the human personality thus:

> Since the mind and the soul find expression through the body, both mental and spiritual vigor are in great degree dependent upon physical strength and activity; whatever promotes physical health, promotes the development of a strong mind and a well-balanced character. Without health, no one can as distinctly understand or as completely fulfill his obligations to himself, to his fellow beings, or to his Creator. Therefore the health should be as faithfully guarded as the character.[8]

In that paragraph, we see not only the interrelatedness of mind, body and spirit but also the purpose of living a healthy life—to fulfill man's obligation to himself, to his fellow beings and to his Creator.

Seven Blessed Habits to Radical Wellness proposes a theocentric world view of the pursuit of health. God is the Creator of man and the principles by which he can live a life of wellness. Not only that, God continues to sustain human life every moment, every hour of every day. God is the One who heals man's sicknesses "through the agencies of nature" that are set at work to "restore soundness" to his body.[9]

[6]J.B. Wong, *Christian Wholism: Theological and Ethical Implications in the Postmodern World* (Lanham, MD: University Press of America, 2002), p. IX.
[7]Ángel M. Rodriguez, "The health-reform program contributes to manifest God's loving concern for humankind," *Perspective Digest*, https://1ref.us/1ee (accessed May 5, 2020).
[8]Ellen G. White, *Education* (Mountain View, CA: Pacific Press, 1903), p. 195.
[9]Ellen G. White, *The Ministry of Healing* (Mountain View, CA: Pacific Press, 1905), p. 112.

To consider the centrality of spirituality in better living is to recognize the true nature and purpose of human life. When this is done, the stage is set for a deeply fulfilling experience. In each of us can then be fulfilled the apostle John's wish for his friend Gaius when he wrote to him thus: "Beloved, I pray that you may prosper in all things and be in health, just as your soul prospers" (3 John 2).

As Dr. Lorraine Day aptly wrote: "Simply put, the process of getting well is the process of getting to know God."[10]

The handle that *Seven Blessed Habits to Radical Wellness* uses to get a grasp of the full spectrum of human health and wellness is the GARDENS© integrated model of health promotion and education. GARDENS© is an acronym for the foundational principles of total health and wellness found in the Bible. It is an integrative, wholistic, theocentric, gospel-centered and evidence-based model of health promotion and education, elaborated and defined as follows:[11]

God — The Source and Sustainer …
Atmosphere — The Cradle and Environment …
Relationships — The Meaning and Fulfillment …
Decisions — The Direction and Destiny …
Exercise — The Function and Purpose …
Nutrition — The Nourishment and Sustenance …
Salvation — The Restoration and Perpetuation …
… of Life, Health, and Happiness.

Each of the seven elements of this model has a practical application. The practical application of these principles is the focus of this book.

---

[10]Lorraine Day, *You Can't Improve on God* (Thousand Palms, CA: Rockford Press, 1997), p. 26.
[11]The GARDENS© integrated model of health promotion and education was formulated by Libni A. Cerdenio as the framework for the wholistic health teaching ministry of Wellness Plus Institute.

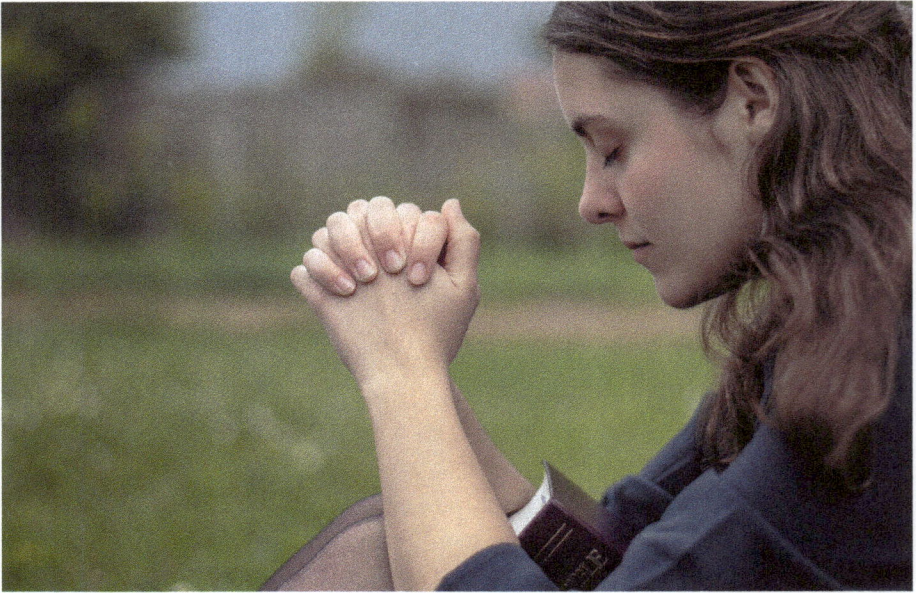

Chapter 1

Pray Fervently to God Always

Blessed Wellness Habit Number 1

There is in the heart of every human being a deep hunger for connection with God that makes everyone prone to pray. God Himself put that hunger there for our good. The wise King Solomon said, "[God] has also set eternity in the human heart" (Eccles. 3:11, NIV).

In his *Confessions*, Book I, Augustine of Hippo (AD 354–430) affirmed King Solomon's words when he wrote: "For Thou hast made us for Thyself and our hearts are restless till they rest in Thee."[12]

In *Pensees*, a collection of his writings, the French physicist and philosopher Blaise Pascal (1623–1662) concurred with King Solomon and St. Augustine: "There is a God-shaped vacuum in the heart of each man

---

[12]"*Confessions* (Augustine)," Wikipedia, https://1ref.us/1ef (accessed May 7, 2020).

which cannot be satisfied by any created thing but only by God the Creator, made known through Jesus Christ."[13]

More recently, Tim Clinton and Max Davis echoed Pascal's words thus:

> There's a sin-gouged hole in the heart of every person alive—a deep void that screams to be filled. We attempt to fill that void with everything from adrenalin rushing activities to relationships to careers. But the problem with these attempts is this: none of them will ultimately satisfy. Oh, you may find a certain amount of enjoyment and even contentment in those things for a while, but in the end they will leave you empty, longing for something more.[14]

❀❀❀❀

Prayer is a must to experience radical wellness. "It is a part of God's plan to grant us, in answer to the prayer of faith, that which He would not bestow did we not thus ask."[15]

> [One day,] there was a woman who had had a discharge of blood for twelve years, and though she had spent all her living on physicians, she could not be healed by anyone. She came up behind him [Jesus Christ] and touched the fringe of his garment, and immediately her discharge of blood ceased. And Jesus said, "Who was it that touched me?" When all denied it, Peter said, "Master, the crowds surround you and are pressing in on you!" But Jesus said, "Someone touched me, for I perceive that power has gone out from me." And when the woman saw that she was not hidden, she came trembling, and falling down before him declared in the presence of all the people why she had touched him, and how she had been immediately healed. And he said to her, "Daughter, your faith has made you well; go in peace." (Luke 8:43–48, ESV)

That healing power from Jesus Christ still flows to those who come to Him through prayer today.

One Saturday afternoon many years ago, I was so overwhelmed with anger at some people in my office who I believed were framing me up for

---

[13]B. Pascal, *Pensées* (New York, NY: Penguin Books, 1966), p. 75.
[14]Tim Clinton and Max Davis, "Only God Can Fill the Void," DR. JAMES DOBSON'S family talk, https://1ref.us/1eg (accessed May 5, 2020).
[15]Ellen G. White, *Prayer* (Nampa, ID: Pacific Press, 2002), p. 47.

failure. I knelt down beside my bed and unburdened myself to God in prayer in the name of Jesus. Before I even got up, I felt the heavy burden lifted away from me. The anger and hostility flew away. Jesus, my Savior and Lord, healed me that day. Praise God!

As a Man in Palestine, Jesus Christ's persona attracted so much attention from people far and near. Word about the amazing truths He taught and the miracles He did spread like the sweet scent of myrrh refreshing the countryside.

His soothing, calming character swept hopelessness away. "And wherever he came, in villages, cities, or countryside, they laid the sick in the marketplaces and implored him that they might touch even the fringe of his garment. And as many as touched it were made well" (Mark 6:56, ESV).

Even foreigners (non-Jews) were awed by and believed in Him. Consider this story about a Roman centurion (a commander of 100 soldiers) who brought his sick servant to Jesus:

> Now a centurion had a servant who was sick and at the point of death, who was highly valued by him. When the centurion heard about Jesus, he sent to him elders of the Jews, asking him to come and heal his servant. And when they came to Jesus, they pleaded with him earnestly, saying, "He is worthy to have you do this for him, for he loves our nation, and he is the one who built us our synagogue." And Jesus went with them. When he was not far from the house, the centurion sent friends, saying to him, "Lord, do not trouble yourself, for I am not worthy to have you come under my roof. Therefore, I did not presume to come to you. But say the word, and let my servant be healed. For I too am a man set under authority, with soldiers under me: and I say to one, 'Go,' and he goes; and to another, 'Come,' and he comes; and to my servant, 'Do this,' and he does it." When Jesus heard these things, he marveled at him, and turning to the crowd that followed him, said, "I tell you, not even in Israel have I found such faith." And when those who had been sent returned to the house, they found the servant well. (Luke 7:2–10, ESV)

Evidently, this Roman commander told his servant about this wonderful Man called Jesus. I presume the servant believed his master. More than that, other people interceded for the centurion and his servant. The Jewish leaders told Him that the centurion was "worthy to have you do this for him, for he loves our nation, and he is the one who built us our synagogue."

As the story goes, Jesus healed the servant, seemingly through and by the master and religious leaders' intercession. Although Jesus did not need them to heal the servant, He honored their intercessory faith. This story shows how Jesus Christ honors and accedes to friend's and family's faithful prayers for their loved ones.

Thank God for godly friends and loved ones who never cease to pray in our behalf.

While in the seminary, I went through a serious episode of doubt about the nature of Jesus Christ. It was a dangerous situation because the Bible says, "Believe in the Lord Jesus, and you will be saved, you and your household" (Acts 16:31, ESV). And "Whoever believes in the Son has eternal life; whoever does not obey the Son shall not see life, but the wrath of God remains on him (John 3:36, ESV).

It affected me so much that I could not help but go to my very spiritual major professor (a professor who is a seminary student's advisor in his major course of study, which in my case was systematic theology) to talk about it. I saw Dr. Norman Gulley in his home office. After some time of confession and counseling, he prayed with and for me. As he was praying, I felt a warm current flowing from my crown to the soles of my feet. And after we prayed, all the doubt in my mind left me. Jesus Christ through the Holy Spirit healed my spiritual malady through the intercession of my professor. Praise be to Him!

A few years ago, I found a book entitled *Incredible Answers to Prayer*. The author, Roger Morneau, was a salesman who dedicated his life to prayer ministry. The book is an account of some of his experiences of answered intercessory prayers.

I was so inspired reading about a dying man who was healed from heart disease, a rebellious son who was reconciled with his parents, a couple whose rocky relationship was saved from divorce and many more incredible answers to Morneau's fervent prayers.

I was the RN QI coordinator of a rehabilitation and care center when I was reading Morneau's book. Deep in my heart, I longed for such an experience of God's favor manifested by answered intercessory prayers.

One day, as I was leaving my office, the Assistant Director of Nursing (ADON) accosted me with a special consultation request. She briefed me about one particular problem patient—an elderly man who was combative and who had fallen out of bed multiple times. She told me that the nurses had done everything within their scope of practice to no avail. As we parted, I assured her that since the staff had done everything they could do, I could just do one more thing—pray for her (the ADON), the patient, the nurses and other caregivers.

Before I left the parking lot, I paused and sent a heartfelt petition to God on the patient and his caregivers' behalf. The next morning—and throughout that week—I stealthily walked by the patient's room to see how he was doing. I was thrilled to know that he was no longer combative and falling off the bed. In fact, I would often see him sleeping quietly as I passed by.

Quite incredulous about what I was seeing, I would purposely read his chart every day. I always looked for either doctors' or nurses' notes that would show any new medications ordered and given, or nursing interventions done. But I found none.

To this day, I praise the Lord for the privilege of praying for a fellow human being in need of Jesus Christ's healing power.

❀ ❀ ❀ ❀

One vivid memory I have growing up is that of waking up in the middle of the night to see the silhouettes of my father and mother kneeling down together in prayer. I could overhear them fervently interceding for me and my siblings.

I grew up in such a home where prayer was said during morning worship, at breakfast, lunch, dinner and during evening worship as well. I even remember my father praying before he and I would take a bath at the spring by the hillside where we drew water for our drinking and cooking needs. From an early age, prayer has been part of my daily routine. It has enriched my life as I have gone through the many milestones in my journey.

One example of how prayer has enriched my life came back to my consciousness while I was doing my devotional reading recently. I came across the following passage that moved and inspired me so much: "Nothing that in any way concerns our peace is too small for Him [God] to notice."[16] Reading that quote brought me back to an unforgettable experience when I was just three months into my immigrant life in the USA.

My family and I lived in the small town of Pecos in the great southwest of Texas where my wife Beth worked as a nurse at the Reeves

---

[16]Ellen G. White, *Steps to Christ* (Mountain View, CA: Pacific Press, 1892), p. 100.

County Hospital. I was looking for but could not find a job. All my prospective employers either said, "You have no US experience," or "You are overqualified." The publisher of the *Pecos Enterprise*—the county newspaper—told me, "You are a little late; I just hired a new managing editor last week."

After three months of seeking and not finding a job, I yielded to my wife's suggestion that I get educated and trained as a nurse. So, I enrolled in the closest school—more than fifty miles away—Odessa College's extension vocational nursing program at the Winkler County Memorial Hospital in Kermit, Texas.

The science subjects were a little difficult for me to study at first, being a liberal arts college graduate and having been away from school for more than a decade. But I was able to think of and implement a personal study strategy that made me the highest scorer in our classes' first written exam. My classmates, half who were Hispanic and half were white, were impressed. They elected me their class president.

One day I presided over a meeting where we decided to contribute a dollar each as a token of our sympathy to a classmate whose mother had died. We set a deadline for giving our contributions. But when the deadline came, I had no dollar to give. Being a new immigrant in the USA and not yet fully acculturated, I was in an emotional dilemma. I was still ingrained in the Filipino value of *hiya* (shame). I dared not borrow money from any of my classmates.

In my despondency, I silently prayed, "God, if You are there, please help me with my problem. I need to give a dollar to my classmate, but I only have ninety cents in my pocket."

After I said that prayer, I went out of the hospital and walked along the parking spaces just outside the hospital entrance. I was looking for perchance a quarter or so on the ground. But I saw none. I reached the end of the parking lot and turned around. On my way back, a flash came from one of the empty spaces. As I came and looked closer on the ground, lo and behold there was a brightly shining dime reflecting the rays of the summer sun. The dime had neither any scratch nor dirt—like it just came from the mint! The hairs on my body stood as I realized God heard and answered my prayer.

This experience was very significant to me because for some time I had been feeling guilty for leaving the job God had given me in the Philippines.

But when God heard and answered my prayer in Kermit, Texas, I felt God was telling me, "It's OK, Libni, even if you left the job I prepared for and gave you in the Philippines, I still love you. We can still work together even here in the US." (Unknown to me at that time, God was preparing me for my health and wellness ministry and advocacy today.)

To this day, I am amazed at how God made sure that I knew He heard and answered my simple prayer. For if my guardian angel put the dime on the ground during my first pass, I would forever be thinking it was just a coincidence. But as it happened, I know God did hear and answer my prayer!

☘☘☘☘

What is prayer, and how does it impact our lives?

One day in the early nineties, a friend persuaded me to buy a satellite dish receiver from his networking company. We set it up on the roof of our house. After reading the instructions, we set ourselves to do it. After some time and effort, we were able to position the antenna as it should be. The television set in our living room came alive with intelligible sounds and colorful images. My family and I were then able to watch TV programs that we chose and enjoyed.

> *Prayer puts us in sync with the will and purposes of God—the Source, Sustainer and Healer of our life, health and happiness.*

In a sense, that is how prayer works. Prayer puts us in sync with the will and purposes of God—the Source, Sustainer and Healer of our life, health and happiness.

Prayer does not change God. As the communication satellite remains geostationary, so is God "the same yesterday and today and forever" (Heb. 13:8). Prayer changes us. It opens the door for us to a healthy, happy and holy life—just the way God intended human life to be from the very beginning.

Don't block your prayers. One day, my wife Beth and I attended a seminar on estate planning held by a law firm close to where we live. We learned some introductory knowledge on establishing a living trust. We learned that we can protect our assets from perceived future threats due to beneficiaries who may not be able to use their inheritance wisely. Examples given were beneficiaries who may be into unhealthy behaviors—like addiction to dangerous drugs—that may jeopardize the good intentions we have for the use of the assets we would like to leave to our chosen beneficiaries. By giving specific instructions as to the use of the bequeathed assets, we can be sure the legacy we leave behind will not be wasted.

This thought takes us to one key condition to a meaningful prayer life: "The Lord will not hear us if we hold on to any known sin. But He always hears the prayers of a person who is sorry for sin."[17]

The Bible is very straightforward about this subject. "If I regard iniquity in my heart, the Lord will not hear" (Ps. 66:18). In His parabolic teaching on entering into the narrow gate, Jesus said that there are people professing to know Him who will be turned away from entering into His kingdom. He will tell them, "'Depart from Me, all you workers of iniquity'" (Luke 13:27).

Simply, praying to God while harboring darling sins is blocking the blessings of heaven from your life. Will a father give the keys to a $300,000 Bugatti Veyron to his son who always wrecks any car he drives? I think not.

"When all known wrongs are made right, we may believe that God will answer our prayers. Our own goodness will never cause God to love us. It is the goodness of Jesus that will save us; it is His blood that will make us clean."[18]

This is a very important principle to remember. Consider these words when God does not answer prayers for healing:

> I saw that the reason why God did not hear the prayers of His servants for the sick among us more fully was, that He could not be glorified in so doing while they were violating the laws of health. And I also saw that He designed the health reform … to prepare the way for the prayer of faith to be fully answered. Faith and good works should go hand in hand in relieving the afflicted among us, and in fitting them to glorify God here, and to be saved at the coming of Christ.
>
> Many have expected that God would keep them from sickness merely because they have asked Him to do so. But God did not regard their prayers, because their faith was not made perfect by works. God will not work a miracle to keep those from sickness who have no care for themselves, but are continually violating the laws of health, and make no efforts to prevent disease. When we

---

[17]Ellen G. White, "Steps to Jesus," EGW Writings, https://1ref.us/1eh (accessed June 23, 2020).
[18]White, "Steps to Jesus."

do all we can on our part to have health, then may we expect that the blessed results will follow, and we can ask God in faith to bless our efforts for the preservation of health. He will then answer our prayer, if His name can be glorified thereby. But let all understand that they have a work to do. God will not work in a miraculous manner to preserve the health of persons who are taking a sure course to make themselves sick, by their careless inattention to the laws of health.[19]

I can think of no other words to close this chapter than these:

Keep your wants, your joys, your sorrows, your cares, and your fears, before God. You cannot burden Him; you cannot weary Him. He who numbers the hairs of your head is not indifferent to the wants of His children …. "The Lord is very pitiful, and of tender mercy." James 5:11. His heart of love is touched by our sorrows and even by our utterances of them. Take to Him everything that perplexes the mind. Nothing is too great for Him to bear, for He holds up worlds, He rules over all the affairs of the universe. Nothing that in any way concerns our peace is too small for Him to notice. There is no chapter in our experience too dark for Him to read; there is no perplexity too difficult for Him to unravel. No calamity can befall the least of His children, no anxiety harass the soul, no joy cheer, no sincere prayer escape the lips, of which our heavenly Father is unobservant, or in which He takes no immediate interest. "He healeth the broken in heart, and bindeth up their wounds." Psalm 147:3. The relations between God and each soul are as distinct and full as though there were not another soul upon the earth to share His watchcare, not another soul for whom He gave His beloved Son.[20]

Pray fervently to receive God's gift of radical wellness. He loves to see us well!

---

[19]Ellen G. White, *Counsels on Diet and Foods* (Washington, DC: Review and Herald, 1938), pp. 25–26.
[20]Ellen G. White, *Steps to Christ* (Mountain View, CA: Pacific Press, 1892), p. 100.

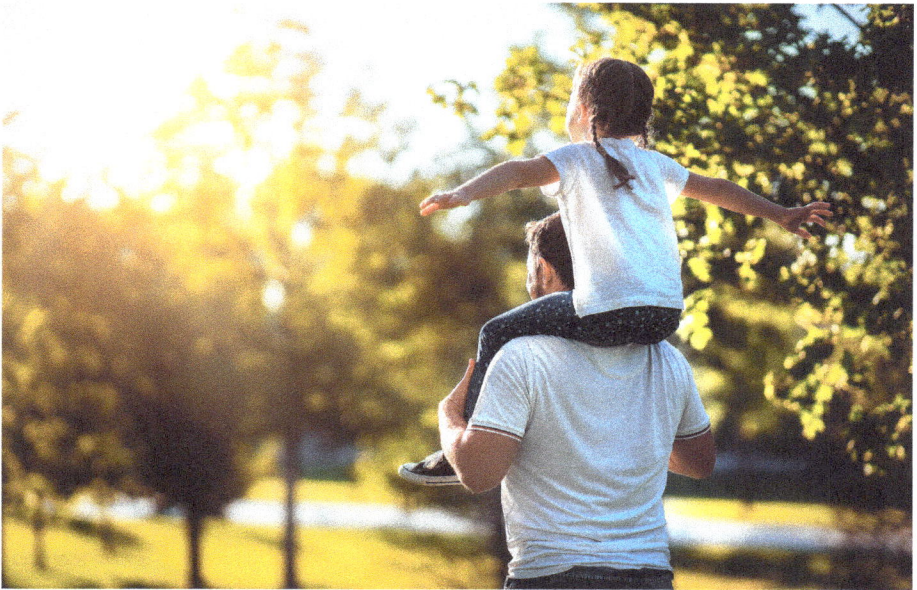

Chapter 2

Embrace All God's Gifts with Gratitude

Blessed Wellness Habit Number 2

W hen I was in college, someone gave a small group of my friends and I an informal but interesting quiz. We were given a list with a dozen things to choose from, but we were only allowed to have seven items with us if we were anticipating being stranded on the moon. Although the situation given was a hypothetical one, our answers would show the level of critical thinking we had at that stage in life.

"What will it take to live on the moon?" That is the title of an online article that explores the possibility of humans inhabiting the moon and making it a launching pad for further explorations in space.[21] Even without reading the article, we can conclude that it is a hard question to answer given the harsh lunar environment. It just isn't fit for human beings to survive there.

Have you heard about the "rule of threes" for human survival? Here they are: (1) You can survive only three minutes without breathable air. (2) You can survive only three hours in a harsh environment (extreme heat or cold). (3) You can survive only three days without drinkable water. (4) You can survive only three weeks without food.[22]

The Creation record enumerates God's amazing gifts for human survival on planet earth:

> In the beginning God created the heavens and the earth. The earth was without form, and void; and darkness *was* on the face of the deep. And the Spirit of God was hovering over the face of the waters. Then God said, "Let there be light" …. a firmament …. dry *land* …. grass … herb[s] … fruit tree[s] …. lights in the firmament …. sea creatures … bird[s] …. beast[s] of the earth …. Then God saw everything that He had made, and indeed *it was* very good. (Gen. 1:1–31)

If you noticed, in this narrative God was like an expectant parent preparing for the birth of the progenitors of the human race. Before He could create human life, God created a suitable cradle and environment for that life which needed not only to survive but also to blossom and flourish.

God gave me this insight when I reread the Creation story once again as my wife and I were expecting the birth of our firstborn. We had to have a crib, clothes, diapers, baby food and everything else our new baby needed to live comfortably.

During Creation, we see God manifesting not only His omnipotent and creative power to bring life into this world, but also His pure and perfect character of love toward His creatures. It reveals His purpose and design for our existence. We were created not to endure life but to enjoy it.

The atmosphere was good. Everything that God designed at Creation was good. The dynamic interrelationship of the components of the earth's atmosphere established at Creation is what continues to support and

---

[21]Todd Bates, "What will it take to live on the moon?" Phys.org, https://1ref.us/1ei (accessed May 5, 2020).

[22]"Rule of threes (survival)," Wikipedia, https://1ref.us/1ej (accessed May 5, 2020).

promote life on earth. What are the components in our good atmosphere and the implications of that goodness to us?

Air. Air is integral to the existence of life. Without air, any human, animal or plant will soon die. Breathed air carries oxygen. If there's oxygen, there's life.

Our atmosphere has a high percentage of oxygen—about twenty-one percent. The rest is nitrogen (seventy-eight percent) and other trace gases. The percentage of oxygen in the air we breathe is very precisely determined. Could there have been life if the percentages had been different? Michael Denton writes on this point:

> Could your atmosphere contain more oxygen and still support life? No! Oxygen is a very reactive element. Even the current percentage of oxygen in the atmosphere, 21 percent, is close to the upper limit of safety for life at ambient temperatures. The probability of a forest fire being ignited increases by as much as 70 percent for every 1 percent increase in the percentage of oxygen in the atmosphere .... the atmosphere is in a state of equilibrium in which risk and benefit are nicely balanced.[23]

More than that, consider the following:

> ... the density, viscosity, and pressure of air are just right. Were it higher, breathing would be as difficult as drawing honey into a needle. Someone might say 'That's easy to fix. We'll just make the hole of the needle larger to increase the rate of flow.' But if we did that in the case of the capillaries in the lungs, the result would be to reduce the size of the area in contact with air, with the result that less oxygen and carbon dioxide would be exchanged in the same amount of time and the respiratory needs of the body would not be satisfied. In other words, the individual values of air's density, viscosity and pressure must all fall within certain limits in order for it to be breathable and those of the air we breathe do exactly that.[24]

In other words, the order God set at Creation needed no improvement because it was very good.

Sunlight. The sun is the driving force behind all our weather and climate. The food we eat exists because of sunlight falling on green plants. Clouds reflect some of the sunlight, reducing the heating of the ground.

[23]G. Gamow, *The Creation of the Universe* (New York, NY: Dover Publications, 1952), p. 95.
[24]Gamow, *Creation*, p. 98.

The atmosphere delays escape of heat to outer space, keeping the ground warm. Sunlight also evaporates water from the oceans, lakes, rivers and plants, humidifying the air.

The right amount of sunlight can have mood-lifting benefits. Exposure to sunlight increases the brain's release of serotonin, a hormone associated with boosting mood and helping a person feel calm and focused. Darker lighting triggers the brain to make another hormone called melatonin, the hormone responsible for helping you sleep. "Low levels of serotonin are associated with a higher risk of major depression with seasonal pattern (formerly known as seasonal affective disorder or SAD). This is a form of depression triggered by the changing seasons."[25] Sunshine is very import-ant in processing Vitamin D in the body.[26]

Water. Water is essential for health and basic survival because it con-stitutes a major portion of the human body.[27] Drinking water does more than just quench our thirst—it's essential to keeping our body function-ing properly and feeling healthy. Nearly all of our body's major systems depend on water to function and survive. Staying hydrated is vital to the healthy functioning of our body.[28]

More than seventy percent of the earth's surface is water. Life on earth is dependent on the availability, distribution, movement and composition of water. The "standard" 70-kilogram (154-pound) male has 60% of his total body weight, or 42 kilograms (92.4 pounds), in the form of water.[29] Significant amounts of water are in all plants and animals. And many spe-cies of plants and animals live in water. The vital body functions cannot happen in the absence of water. Water is what God designed as a beverage for man, plants and animals. Water helps flush poisons—byproducts of vital life processes—from the body and gives life to every cell.

Water has a very simple atomic structure. This structure consists of two hydrogen atoms bonded to one oxygen atom. The nature of the atomic structure of water causes its molecules to have unique

[25]Rachel Nall, "What Are the Benefits of Sunlight?" healthline, https://1ref.us/1ek (accessed May 11, 2020).

[26]Jacob Terranova, "The Sunshine Supplement: Understanding Vitamin D and the Sun," THORNE, https://1ref.us/1el (accessed May 11, 2020).

[27]"The Water in You: Water and the Human Body," USGS, https://1ref.us/1em (accessed May 11, 2020).

[28]"Water: Essential to your body," MAYO CLINIC HEALTH SYSTEM, https://1ref.us/1en (accessed May 11, 2020).

[29]D. Silverthorn, et al. *Human Physiology, an Integrated Approach* (fourth edition) (San Francisco, CA: Pearson Benjamin Cummings, 2009), p. 154.

electrochemical properties. The hydrogen side of the water molecule has a slight positive charge. On the other side of the molecule a negative charge exists. This molecular polarity causes water to be a powerful solvent and is responsible for its strong surface tension.[30]

"[I]f [the water polarity is] greater: heat of fusion and vaporization would be too great for life to exist; if smaller the heat of fusion and vaporization would be too small for life's existence; liquid water would become too inferior a solvent for life chemistry to proceed; ice would not float, leading to a runaway freeze-up."[31] Is this not proof of how God fine-tuned the atmosphere so that it could support life?

Land. Just imagine if all the earth's surface was water. Where would the majestic redwoods grow? How could we enjoy the succulent and fresh tropical fruits? Where could we find meadows of bright shining flowers? Where would the birds and fowls roost? Where would we run around just for fun and frolic? Indeed, the sunlight, air, water and dry land combination God made on Creation week was very good.

The land provides healthful benefits. A novel concept known as grounding or earthing is when someone goes barefoot in dirt, grass, or water. Nobel Prize winner Richard Feynman claimed that "grounding equalized the electronic potential between the body and the earth, so the body becomes an extension of the earth's magnetic field. This potential 'cancels, reduces, and pushes away electrical fields from the body.'" Grounding is also thought to improve sleep, pain management, stress, inflammation and immunity.[32]

The spiritual atmosphere was good. In the beginning, not only the physical environment on earth was conducive to human life. The spiritual atmosphere was also very good. I have not yet found a better exposition on how Adam and Eve must have perceived the meaning of everything they saw on the very first day of their lives as the following:

"'God is love'… [was] written upon every opening bud, upon every spire of springing grass. The lovely birds making the air vocal with their happy songs, the delicately tinted flowers in their perfection perfuming the air, the lofty trees of the forest with their rich foliage of living green—all

---

[30]"Physical Properties of Water," Physical Geography, https://1ref.us/1eo (accessed May 11, 2020).

[31]Anthony Walsh, *Answering the New Atheists: How Science Points to God and to the Benefits of Christianity* (Wilmington, DE: Vernon Press, 2019), p. 87.

[32]David Brady, "Health Benefits of Grounding (Earthing)," The Fibro Fix, https://1ref.us/1ep (accessed May 11, 2020).

… [testified] to the tender fatherly care of … God, and to His desire to make His children happy."[33]

After He created Adam and Eve, God rested on the seventh day of Creation week. In other words, the human progenitor's first day of life was spent in companionship and communion with their Creator. To understand this from today's point of view, it is just like a father and mother taking time off on a paternity/maternity leave to attend the birth of their child. No one can miss that day—the parents' celebration of joy and love on the arrival and entrance of their baby into their lives. The parents' first day with their baby is a manifestation of their commitment to love, cherish and care for him all his life. The Creator's first day with Adam and Eve expressed His delight at their arrival. It was an expression of His covenant to love, care for and sustain the race that He had brought into existence in the world.

> *After He created Adam and Eve, God rested on the seventh day of Creation week. In other words, the human progenitor's first day of life was spent in companionship and communion with their Creator.*

As every child's birthday should remind him of his parents' lifelong commitment to love, cherish and support him, so should every seventh day remind people of God's enduring love for man. This injunction from the Bible is certainly apropos to a generation who has virtually forgotten God:

Keep in memory the Sabbath and let it be a holy day. On six days do all your work: But the seventh day is a Sabbath to the Lord your God; on that day you are to do no work, you or your son or your daughter, your man-servant or your woman-servant, your cattle or the man from a strange country who is living among you: For in six days the Lord made heaven and earth, and the sea, and everything in them, and he took his rest on the seventh day: for this reason the Lord has given his blessing to the seventh day and made it holy. (Exod. 20:8–7, BBE)

---

[33]Ellen G. White, *Steps to Christ* (Mountain View, CA: Pacific Press, 1892), p. 10.

The seventh-day Sabbath was meant to be a blessing to man. As Jesus Himself said, "The Sabbath was made for man, not man for the Sabbath" (Mark 2:27, ESV). More than just being a memorial and celebration of Creation, the weekly Sabbath is also a reminder of God's acts to effect man's salvation.

In Exodus 20:2, BBE, God said this to the children of Israel before declaring His Ten Commandments: "I am the Lord your God who took you out of the land of Egypt, out of the prison-house." Then, in the New Testament book of Hebrews, the writer points to the seventh-day Sabbath as a reference in expounding on the salvation rest that is available to everyone who believes in God's salvation plan for man as manifested in the life, ministry, death on the cross and resurrection of Jesus Christ.

> Let us then, though we still have God's word that we may come into his rest, go in fear that some of you may be unable to do so. And, truly, the good news came to us, even as it did to them; but the hearing of the word did them no good, because they were not united in faith with the true hearers. For those of us who have belief come into his rest; even as he has said, As I said in my oath when I was angry, They may not come into my rest: though the works were done from the time of the making of the world. For in one place he has said of the seventh day, And God had rest from all his works on the seventh day; and in the same place he says again, They will not come into my rest. So that as it is clear that some have to go in, and that the first hearers of the good news were not able to go in because they went against God's orders, after a long time, again naming a certain day, he says in David, Today (as he had said before), Today if you will let his voice come to your ears, be not hard of heart, for if Joshua had given them rest, he would not have said anything about another day. So that there is still a Sabbath-keeping for the people of God. For the man who comes into his rest has had rest from his works, as God did from his. (Heb. 4:1–10, BBE)

More than God's message of love through the natural atmosphere and the seventh-day Sabbath, God has provided an even better and clearer "atmosphere" of goodness around this world. "For God had such love for the world that he gave his only Son, so that whoever has faith in him may not come to destruction but have eternal life. God did not send his

Son into the world to be judge of the world; he sent him so that the world might have salvation through him" (John 3:16–17, BBE).

Science says that we need at least four basic elements to survive: air, water, food and light. And look at what our Lord Jesus Christ said about Himself: He is the living water (John 4:10–14), He is "the breath of life" (Gen. 2:7; John 5:26), "I am the light of the world" (John 8:12) and "I am the bread of life" (John 6:35).

It is no wonder that the inspired writer wrote: "In the matchless gift of His son, God has encircled the whole world with an atmosphere of grace as real as the air which circulates around the globe. All who choose to breathe this life-giving atmosphere will live, and grow up to the stature of men and women in Christ Jesus."[34]

We usually take the life-friendly atmosphere we have on planet earth for granted—an abundance of air, sunshine, water and food. We never think about being grateful for it to the One who created and sustains it so we can not only survive but thrive on this our only home sweet home in the vastness of the cosmos.

To embrace God's gifts means to have an attitude of gratitude and praise to God for creating us. Like the psalmist, we ought to say: "I will praise You, for I am fearfully *and* wonderfully made; marvelous are Your works, *and* that my soul knows very well" (Ps. 139:14).

The Harvard Medical School reported that "In positive psychology research, gratitude is strongly and consistently associated with greater happiness. *Gratitude helps people feel more positive emotions, relish good experiences, improve their health,* deal with adversity, and build strong relationships."[35]

Definitely, embracing all God's gifts with gratitude is essential to radical wellness.

---

[34]Ellen G. White, *God's Amazing Grace* (Hagerstown, MD: Review and Herald, 1973), p. 238.
[35]"Giving thanks can make you happier," Harvard Health Publishing, https://1ref.us/1eq (accessed May 11, 2020), (emphasis added).

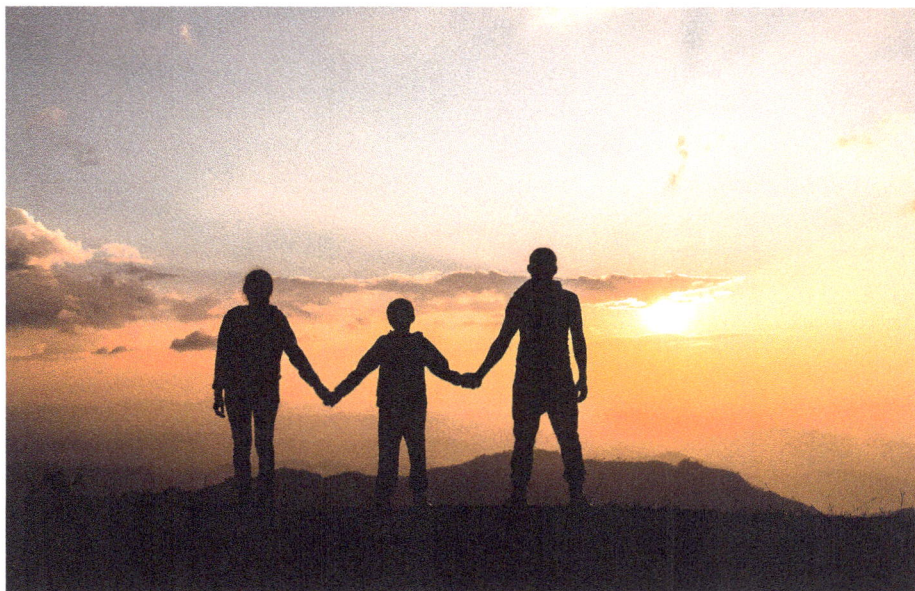

Chapter 3

Love Unconditionally as God Does

Blessed Wellness Habit Number 3

Normally, I would have been excited to go home. But that partic-ular day, it was different. I did not want to leave my office at Philippine Publishing House. Since my wife went to visit her parents for a vacation with our two toddler boys, coming home was like entering into a dark, eerie cave. It was our first time to be separated after getting married. It was my first stark encounter with life sans my loved ones around.

Another time, my teenage daughter, who was at the stage where she felt she had to have a boyfriend, called me from Texas and jokingly said she needed some "inspiration" to get through this especially difficult week in college. Beyond her banter, I could sense her new discovery that life without significant relationships is quite empty and meaningless.

God created man a relational being. He created him with three levels of relationships.

The first level is man's relationship with God Himself. This human relatedness to God is the deep and profound meaning of God resting on the seventh day of Creation week. Like human parents at the birth of their child, God took a day off to spend quality time with His children. It is in that context that God likes man to call the seventh-day Sabbath a delight. "If you keep the Sabbath with care, not doing your business on my holy day; and if the Sabbath seems to you a delight, ... Then the Lord will be your delight; and I will put you on the high places of the earth; ... for the mouth of the Lord has said it" (Isa. 58:13–14, BBE).

In entering into God's rest on the Sabbath day, we commune with Him and learn of His great love and care for us.

In the Gospels of Matthew, Mark, Luke and John we see the incarnate God—Jesus Christ—eagerly relating with men: healing the sick, feeding the hungry, helping the poor, teaching the ignorant and preaching to them that "the kingdom of God has come near" (Mark 1:15, NIV). And God Himself said this about the value of man in His eyes: "Are not five sparrows given in exchange for two farthings? and God has every one of them in mind. But even the hairs of your head are numbered. Have no fear: you are of more value than a flock of sparrows" (Luke 12:6–7, BBE).

> *Today, God invites every man, woman and child to enter into His rest—rest from fear, anxiety, hopelessness and sin: "Come to me, all you who are troubled and weighted down with care, and I will give you rest. Take my yoke on you and become like me, for I am gentle and without pride, and you will have rest for your souls; for my yoke is good, and the weight I take up is not hard" (Matt. 11:28–30, BBE).*

Today, God invites every man, woman and child to enter into His rest—rest from fear, anxiety, hopelessness and sin: "Come to me, all you who are troubled and weighted down with care, and I will give you rest. Take my yoke on you and become like me, for I am gentle and without pride, and you will have rest for your souls; for my yoke is good, and the weight I take up is not hard" (Matt. 11:28–30, BBE). In worship of the Creator, in obedience to His commands, and in loving service to his fellow human beings, man shows his allegiance and relatedness to God.

The second level is man's relationship with his fellow human beings. In creating Adam, God knew that he would have this void if he did not feel a connectedness to another human being. So, He created Eve.

> And the Lord God said, It is not good for the man to be by himself: I will make one like himself as a help to him …. And the Lord God sent a deep sleep on the man, and took one of the bones from his side while he was sleeping, joining up the flesh again in its place: And the bone which the Lord God had taken from the man he made into a woman, and took her to the man. And the man said, This is now bone of my bone and flesh of my flesh: let her name be Woman because she was taken out of Man. For this cause will a man go away from his father and his mother and be joined to his wife; and they will be one flesh. (Gen. 2:18, 21–24, BBE)

Adam alone was "not good." On the other hand, Adam becoming "one" with Eve was "very good." Moreover, Adam (male) and Eve (female) were a reflection of God's image in humanity. "And God made man in his image, in the image of God he made him: male and female he made them" (Gen. 1:27, BBE).

The third level of human relatedness that God established was man in relationship to plants and animals—His lower creatures.

> And God said, Let us make man in our image, like us: and let him have rule over the fish of the sea and over the birds of the air and over the cattle and over all the earth and over every living thing which goes flat on the earth …. And God gave them his blessing and said to them … be rulers over the fish of the sea and over the birds of the air and over every living thing moving on the earth. (Gen. 1:26, 28, BBE)

❋❋❋❋

Memory researchers have identified something called "the reminiscence bump." This means that "our strongest memories come from things that happened to us between the ages of 10 and 30."[36]

One memorable moment I remember from that timeline was when one of my high school teachers said that there are three basic ways in which justice is meted out in society: savage, Mosaic and Christian. Savage justice is death for stealing a G-string. Mosaic is "an eye for an eye, a tooth for a tooth" (Exod. 21:24, NLT). And Christian justice is focused on rehabilitation and restoration of the offending individual.

At one time when I recalled this idea, it dawned on me that there are three ways by which human beings base their relationship with one another—savage, Mosaic and Christian. Savage—acceptance by blood and birth. Mosaic—reciprocity necessitated by common needs. Christian—"as I [Christ] have loved you" (John 15:12).

Loving everyone as God loves us is the essence of Christian living. Jesus Christ said, "I give you a new law: Have love one for another; even as I have had love for you, so are you to have love one for another" (John 13:34, BBE). How does He love us erring, sinful mortals? "[M]y love for you is an eternal love" (Jer. 31:3).

Here are a few applications of Christianity's treat-others-as-Christ-has-treated-you motif (See Eph. 4, 5 and 6):

- "Husbands, have love for your wives, *even as Christ had love for the church*, and gave himself for it" (Eph. 5:25, BBE, emphasis added).
- "Wives, be under the authority of your husbands, *as of the Lord*" (Eph. 5:22, BBE, emphasis added).
- "[F]athers, do not make your children angry: but give them training *in the teaching and fear of the Lord*" (Eph. 6:4, BBE, emphasis added).
- "Children, do what is ordered by your fathers and mothers *in the Lord:* for this is right" (Eph. 6:1, BBE, emphasis added).

Who spoiled the golden morning? In the beginning, human relationships were meant to be happy: no less than He who created human relatedness said that it was "very good." However, that is not what we see in the world today. Many times, relationships are a bittersweet experience. After a short honeymoon, the bliss of togetherness begins to fade away.

Believe it or not, the root of brokenness in human relationships emanated from paradise. Like geological faults that may run unseen for miles,

---

[36]Frank T. McAndrew, "Why high school stays with us forever," *The Conversation*, https://1ref.us/1er (accessed May 11, 2020).

they nevertheless continue to threaten our happiness with impending disaster.

When earth's first couple, at the instigation of the evil one, disobeyed God's command in the Garden, all of their levels of relationships became broken. Where before they eagerly anticipated "the sound of the Lord God walking in the garden in the evening wind" (Gen. 3:8, BBE), they now "went to a secret place among the trees of the garden" (Ibid.) to hide from Him. Where before their hearts beat as one, they now pointed fingers at each other, mutually blaming each other for the misfortune they were in (Gen. 3:12–13). Where before they had dominion over the earth, "the earth … [was now] cursed …. Thorns and waste plants … [came] up, and [by] … the hard work of … [their] hands …. [they got their] bread till … [they went] back to the earth from which … [they] were taken: for dust … [they were] and to the dust … [they would] go back" (Gen. 3:17–19, BBE).

Recently, I had to wake my wife Beth up from a bad dream. She said she dreamt that the devil was out to destroy me and that she was going after him.

Let me tell you that it is not a bad dream, but an absolute reality that the evil one is out trying to destroy people today. The apostle Peter counseled the early Christians thus: "Be serious and keep watch; the Evil One, who is against you, goes about like a lion with open mouth in search of food; Do not give way to him but be strong in your faith, in the knowledge that your brothers who are in the world undergo the same troubles" (1 Peter 5:8–9, BBE).

It was the apostle Paul who gave us an insight into the true dynamics of human relationships today. He said that "our fight … [should not be] against flesh and blood, but against authorities and powers, against the world-rulers of this dark night, against the spirits of evil in the heavens" (Eph. 6:12, BBE). The context of this statement is the apostle's counsel that people should love one another and have unity and harmony in the home, church and society. (See Eph. 4, 5 and 6.)

Make no mistake about it. The devil is a mad bull raging to destroy your birthright to a healthy, happy and wholesome life. On the other hand, Jesus Christ came to earth to heal and restore man's brokenness. Expounding on His mission, He declared: "The Spirit of the LORD is upon Me, because He has anointed Me … to heal the brokenhearted" (Luke 4:18).

How are we to fight? When I was a little boy, I thought I could fight the devil David-like one-on-one. I would go around the farm with my bolo (a large knife used in the Philippines), sling shot and iron ring-tipped rod, daring the devil to show himself to me. In the seminary, I learned that the way to do it was to cling to the old rugged cross. When my wife was telling me about her dream, I told her to stop; we prayed and praised God for His loving care and protection over His loved ones.

In his epistle to the Ephesian Christians, apostle Paul delineated a seven-point strategy for fighting the powers that be of spiritual darkness (Eph. 6:14–18). He told them to:

1. Be "clothed with the true word" (Eph. 6:14, BBE).
2. "[P]ut on the breastplate of righteousness" (Ibid.).
3. "Be ready with the good news of peace as shoes on your feet" (Eph. 6:15, BBE).
4. Use "faith as a cover to keep off all the flaming arrows of the Evil One" (Eph. 6:16, BBE).
5. "[T]ake salvation for your head-dress" (Eph. 6:17, BBE).
6. Have "the sword of the Spirit, which is the word of God" (Ibid.).
7. Pray, "making requests at all times in the Spirit, and keeping watch, with strong purpose, in prayer for all the saints" (Eph. 6:18, BBE).

Love. Please make mine forever. Many people are gravely concerned with the dangers posed by today's technological advances on our traditional values. I once read a newspaper column many years ago about technology as the concomitant tool of selfism, a philosophy that puts self and its material needs at the center of reality. According to this mindset, technology must deliver to self what it wants—efficiently, accurately, in the fastest way, without pain. Computers, instant products in disposable containers and pain relievers are a few of the many tools of this mentality.

How does technology and selfism affect human relationships? The newspaper columnist said that selfism is a philosophy of intolerance to errors and mistakes, time and slow, natural processes and pain. And that is what makes it inhuman. Part of being human is to allow time and natural processes to shape our lives. True love and friendship develop over time. Physical, emotional and spiritual growth take time. To be human means having to experience the pain of wounded emotions, disloyalty, rejection, errors and mistakes in our perceptions, judgments and actions. The columnist concluded that the human condition is precisely full of errors and mistakes—mistakes that need to be absorbed and forgiven. Husbands toward wives, wives toward husbands, parents toward children, children toward parents, families toward families.

However, basic human nature nurtured by the technological preciseness is directly opposed to tolerance, forgiveness and acceptance. We would rather dispose of a problematic relationship than mend and renew it. Just like throwing away a used disposable cup.

The beauty of sanctified humanness is the capacity to forgive and forget, to hope and love again, to let wounds be healed and to dispose of errors and mistakes in the ashes of a resurrected and higher state of relationship.

An eighty-year-long study at Harvard University has affirmed that healthy and happy human relationships contribute to a happy and long life.[37]

According to Robert Waldinger, director of the study, "The surprising finding is that our relationships and how happy we are in our relationships has a powerful influence on our health. Taking care of your body is important, but tending to your relationships is a form of self-care too."[38]

God's everlasting love reflected in human relationships is a key component of radical wellness.

Being in happy relationships is healthful; being socially isolated is unhealthy. Chirag Shah, MD, an emergency physician, says: "Chronic loneliness can lead to deterioration in our ability to respond to potential infections as well as the strength of our immune response ...."[39]

God's everlasting love reflected in human relationships is a key component of radical wellness.

---

[37]Liz Mineo, "Good genes are nice, but joy is better," *Harvard Gazette*, https://1ref.us/1es (accessed May 11, 2020).

[38]Mineo, "Good genes."

[39]Kelly Burch, "Loneliness may weaken the immune system — here's how to feel less lonely during social isolation," Insider, https://1ref.us/1et (accessed May 11, 2020).

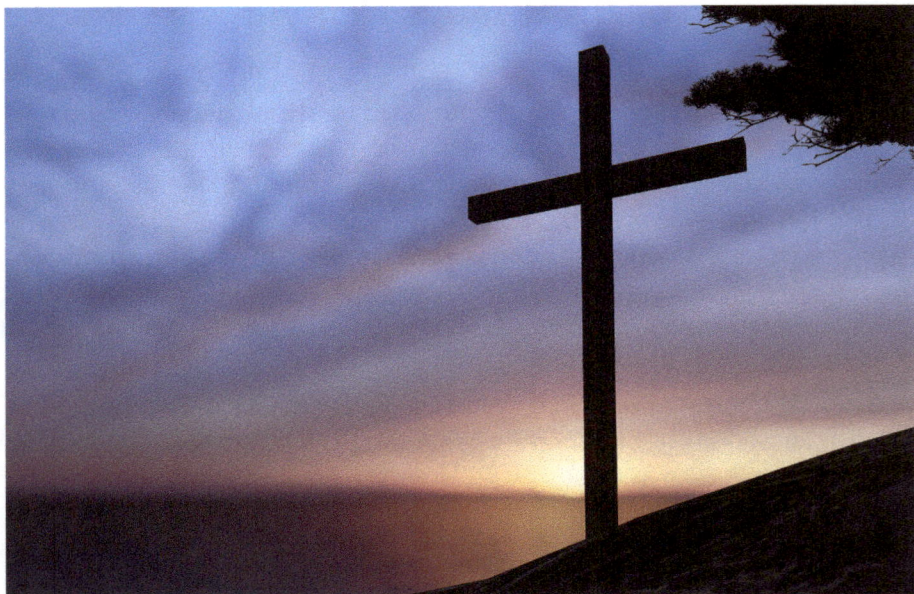

Chapter 4

Follow God's Will for Your Life

Blessed Wellness Habit Number 4

One day, when I was still working as an editor at Philippine Publishing House, my boss—the editor-in-chief—called me into his office. He intimated to me that he had a good plan for me. He wanted me to succeed him as editor-in-chief when he retired. I had no doubt that it would have happened as he planned, except that two weeks after that meeting I gave him my letter of resignation because my family and I were set to immigrate to the USA.

Did you know that the most powerful, loving and beneficent Person in the whole universe has a beautiful plan for your life? Consider this: "'For I know the plans I have for you,' declares the LORD, 'plans to prosper you and not to harm you, plans to give you hope and a future'" (Jer. 29:11, NIV).

Jeremiah 29:11 was actually God's message to the Israelites who were taken captive by Nebuchadnezzar, King of Babylon, when he conquered the Kingdom of Judah. God had purposed for their captivity to last for seventy years. But after that, God promised to bring the captives back to their homeland, rebuild their city (Jerusalem) and restore the Kingdom of Judah. Meanwhile, He told them through the prophet Jeremiah to settle down in Babylon, build houses and plant vineyards while waiting for God's time of restoration. That was the context of that beautiful Bible verse.

Many Bible readers like to apply this verse to themselves. Can we indeed claim it as God's promise to us personally? Russell Moore believes so, but it must be read in context:

> Jeremiah 29:11 must be read in the context of the whole Book of Jeremiah, and the Book of Jeremiah must be read in the context of Israel's story. But then all of Jeremiah and all of Israel's story must be read in the context of God's purposes in Jesus Christ. All the promises of God "find their yes in him" (2 Cor. 1:20). If we are in Christ, then all the horrors of judgment warned about in the prophets have fallen on us, in the cross, where we were united to Christ as he bore the curse of the law (Gal. 3:13). And, if we are in Christ, then all of the blessings promised to Abraham's offspring are now ours, since we are united to the heir of all those promises (Gal. 3:14–29).[40]

It is God's overall plan for all people to accept Jesus Christ into their life. Does God have a specific plan for each of us? How can we know that plan?

One sure way I know is through prayer. If you sincerely pray for God's will for your life, He will show it to you in answer to sincere prayer. I personally experienced God's guidance in my life when I was deciding what major course of study to take when I was in college.

After my sophomore year, I was conflicted in what major courses to take when enrollment time came in June 1973. On one hand, I wanted to take a major in English; on the other hand, I was drawn toward a major in theology. Taking a double major was not feasible for my financial resources.

One day during that summer vacation, I remember pausing to pray by the flagpole on the midpoint along the walkway from the New Administration Building to the Jackson-Sevrens Hall at the then campus of Philippine Union College in Baesa, Caloocan City, Philippines.

[40]Russell Moore, "Does Jeremiah 29:11 Apply to You?" The Gospel Coalition, https://1ref.us/1eu (accessed May 11, 2020).

I petitioned God to guide me in choosing which major course to take. I prayed: "Dear God, please guide me in making my decision; show me what major I need to take, according to Your will and purposes for my life. In Jesus' name I pray. Amen."

Soon two weeks had passed after I uttered that simple prayer. Then I received a letter from the president of the Seventh-day Adventist Church in the Bicol Region of the Philippines. In short, the letter said: "Libni, we would like to help you financially through college, but you need to take the ministerial course." I took that as God's answer to my prayer, loud and clear.

Why God wanted me to major in religion played out during that same school year. The Philippine Publishing House was looking for an editorial intern to be mentored by James Joiner, a missionary who was the editorial consultant there at that time. The one condition was the student to be selected should be taking a religion major. In short, I was selected to fill that vacancy. I was invited to work there on my graduation and served as Associate Editor until I immigrated to the USA with my family in 1986. God hears and answers our prayers. He has blessed me with many of them through the years.

Chris Russell suggests eight principles on how to know God's specific will for your life:

1. *Walk with God.* Seek to know Him, not just about Him. Read His Word, the Bible. Develop a consistent prayer life. Get involved in small Bible study groups. Determine to "Trust in the LORD with all your heart, and lean not on your own understanding; in all your ways acknowledge Him, and He shall direct your paths" (Prov. 3:5–6).
2. *Surrender your will to God's.* "Before God will begin to reveal His will to you, you must be committed to doing whatever it is that He desires for you to do …. Jesus was willing to die for us, so shouldn't we be willing to live for Him?"
3. *Obey what you already know to be God's will.* "If we do not obey the things that God has shown us clearly to be His will, why would we think He would reveal any further information regarding His plan for our lives? Obedience is an important first step."
4. *Seek godly input.* "One key component to finding God's will is to seek the input of godly advisors in your life …. 'Where there is no counsel, the people fall; but in the multitude of counselors there is safety'" (Prov. 11:14).

5. *Pay attention to how God has wired you.* "God has gifted every one of us to perform a special mission for which we alone were created. How amazing is that?"
6. *Listen to God's Spirit.* The author states that he added "a significant component to … [his] prayer life: listening. [T]ake time to listen to what God might have to say to … [you]."
7. *Listen to your heart.* "In addition to listening to the Spirit … [listen also] to your heart. 'Delight yourself also in the LORD, and He shall give you the desires of your heart. Commit your way to the LORD, trust also in Him, and He shall bring it to pass' (Ps. 37:4–5)."
8. *Take a look at your circumstances.* "God often clearly demonstrates His plan for our lives by lining up circumstances in obvious ways. And He also shows us what His will is NOT for us to do in that same way."[41]

So, what is God's plan and purpose for you and me? As far as radical wellness is concerned, I believe God's plan for us is the same as what the apostle John wished his friend Gaius—health and wellness in body, mind and spirit. He wrote: "Dear friend, I hope all is well with you and that you are as healthy in body as you are strong in spirit" (3 John 2, NLT).

The question is: are we willing to follow God's plan for our lives? James Russel Lowell wrote about this issue facing each of us today: "Once to every man and nation comes the moment to decide, in the strife of truth and falsehood, for the good or evil side; some great cause, some new decision, offering each bloom or blight, and the choice goes by forever twixt that darkness and that light."[42]

So, what is God's plan and purpose for you and me? As far as radical wellness is concerned, I believe God's plan for us is the same as what the apostle John wished his friend Gaius—health and wellness in body, mind and spirit. He wrote: "Dear friend, I hope all is well with you and that you are as healthy in body as you are strong in spirit" (3 John 2, NLT).

[41]Chris Russell, "8 Keys to Knowing God's Will For Your Life," Bible Study Tools, https://1ref.us/1ev (accessed May 11, 2020). Note: All portions in quotation are direct quotes.
[42]James Russel Lowell, Quotes.pub, https://1ref.us/1ew (accessed May 11, 2020).

The fact is that every day we choose which side we would like to be on—Christ or His enemy. Obedience to God is the key to the fulfillment of God's beautiful plan for our lives.

> It is those who obey that will be blessed of God. He says that He will bless your children and your lands and all that you lay your hand unto. Do you think that Satan is going to allow this without making a struggle for the mastery?
>
> The enemy is working just as sharply and decidedly now as he worked upon the minds of Adam and Eve in Eden. The people are gathering under his banner, and he is encircling them with his power. But everyone who sees that the law of God is changeless in its character will decide on the side of Christ. If God could have changed one precept of His law to meet the fallen human race, then Jesus Christ need never have come to our earth to die.[43]

This is the challenge for you and me today: "But if you refuse to serve the LORD, then choose today whom you will serve …. But as for me and my family, we will serve the LORD" Josh. 24:15, NLT).

The first new car our family bought when we immigrated to Texas was a Ford Escort, model 1986. It served us well for fourteen years. I remember the first time I tried to fix a problem in that car. I almost broke the rear light housing while trying to change a busted brake light. Then I remembered there was an owner's manual that came with the car. It took me a little time and effort to follow the instructions on how to change a busted brake light, but eventually I was successful.

Desiring to be healthy apart from God's will is like changing a car's busted brake light without consulting the owner's manual. You can end up destroying your health rather than fixing it. God is the ever-loving Guide of our destiny. As in the life of Jeremiah, it is true that: "Before I formed you in the womb I knew you; Before you were born, I sanctified you" (Jer. 1:5).

We need to believe in and accept that gift from God today. God is always at work for our good. A prolific Christian writer emphasized this point when she wrote:

> The Savior in His miracles revealed the power that is continually at work in man's behalf, to sustain and to heal him. Through the agencies of nature, God is working, day by day, hour by hour, moment by moment, to keep us alive, to build up and restore us. When any

[43]Ellen G. White, *Christ Triumphant* (Hagerstown, MD: Review and Herald, 1999), p. 15.

part of the body sustains injury, a healing process is at once begun; nature's agencies are set at work to restore soundness. But the power working through these agencies is the power of God. All life-giving power is from Him. When one recovers from disease, it is God who restores him.[44]

The greatest assurance we have in following God's will for our lives is this: "You will seek me and find me, when you seek me with all your heart" (Jer. 29:13, ESV).

---

[44]Ellen G. White, *The Ministry of Healing* (Mountain View, CA: Pacific Press, 1905), pp. 112–113.

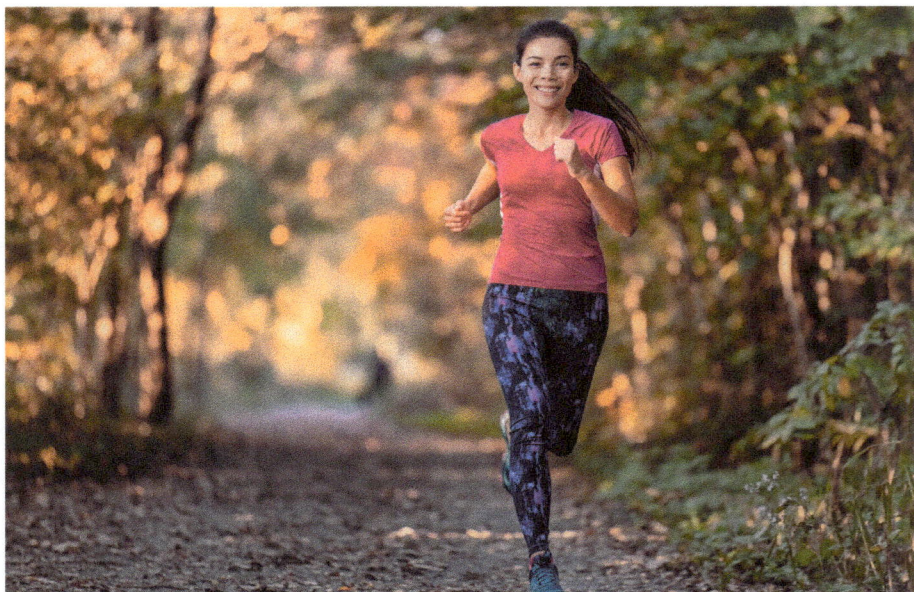

Chapter 5

Just Move It—Body, Mind, and Spirit

Blessed Wellness Habit Number 5

Recently, I read an online article entitled "The Physics of Productivity: Newton's Laws of Getting Stuff Done." In the article, James Clear proposes that "Newton's three laws of motion can be used as an interesting analogy for increasing your productivity, simplifying your work, and improving your life."[45]

For example, Clear suggests that Newton's first law of motion (*"[a]n object either remains at rest or continues to move at a constant*

---

[45]James Clear, "The Physics of Productivity: Newton's Laws of Getting Stuff Done," James Clear, https://1ref.us/1ex (accessed May 11, 2020).

velocity, unless acted upon by an external force"[46]) can be applied as the first law of productivity. "When it comes to being productive, this means one thing: the most important thing is to find a way to get started. Once you get started, it is much easier to stay in motion."[47]

I would like to propose that Newton's first law of motion can also be applied as an analogy for the physics of exercise. Getting started on regular physical, mental and spiritual activities can be the beginning of radical wellness. Motion is an immutable principle of life. The body is designed to move. The health status of all the structures and functions of the body systems are maintained and enhanced by a well-balanced rhythm of purposeful activity and its corollary, adequate rest.

God designed the body to move. In the beginning, God created man for productive activity. It was never His intention that people become a couch potato. "The LORD God placed the man in the Garden of Eden to tend and watch over it" (Gen. 2:15, NLT).

The human anatomy and physiology are designed for motion:

Man's organic structure is made for movement and exercise. Adam and Eve were created to be useful and not idle. They were given the work of tending trees and bushes in the Garden of Eden. Such labor was to call into exercise the wonderful organs of the body. Their happiness was bound up with their labor. "Useful occupation was appointed them as a blessing to STRENGTHEN the BODY, to EXPAND the MIND, and to DEVELOP CHARACTER" (Ed21). The physical powers were to be kept in health by EXERCISE so as to also maintain and strengthen the spiritual powers.[48]

Exercise is necessary to radical wellness; it improves blood circulation throughout the body. "Perfect health depends upon perfect circulation."[49]

"The primary function of the cardiovascular system is the transport of materials to and from all parts of the body. Substances transported by the cardiovascular system can be divided into (1) nutrients, water, and gases that enter the body from the external environment, (2) materials that move

[46]Clear, "Physics."

[47]Clear, "Physics."

[48]Gunther B. Paulien, *The Divine Prescription and Science of Health and Healing* (New York, NY: TEACH Services, Inc, 1995), p. 81.

[49]Ellen G. White, *Healthful Living* (Battle Creek, MI: Medical Missionary Board, 1897), p. 30.

> *Exercise is necessary to radical wellness; it improves blood circulation throughout the body. "Perfect health depends upon perfect circulation."*

from cell to cell within the body, and (3) wastes that the cells eliminate..."[50]

Best exercise practices. What are the criteria for the best exercise practices?

"In creating Adam and Eve, God designed that they should be active and useful."[51]

"As a rule, the exercise most beneficial to the ... [whole person] will be found in useful employment."[52]

An effective exercise program should include the following elements: aerobic exercise; resistance training (weightlifting); flexibility (stretching); and proper nutrition.[53]

Edward R. Laskowski, MD, recommends these exercise guidelines for most healthy adults:

1. **Aerobic activity**. Get at least 150 minutes of moderate aerobic activity or 75 minutes of vigorous aerobic activity a week, or a combination of moderate and vigorous activity. The guidelines suggest that you spread out this exercise during the course of a week.
2. **Strength training**. Do strength training exercises for all major muscle groups at least two times a week. Aim to do a single set of each exercise, using a weight or resistance level heavy enough to tire your muscles after about 12 to 15 repetitions.[54]

So, just do it! Make a decision to exercise and do it! Get an exercise buddy for more chances of sustainability and accountability:

"The most successful fitness partnerships fall into one of three categories: the pal-based buddy system, the small group and the coupled pair .... Workout partners not only get us through a challenging workout, but can help us through life challenges as well."[55]

[50]Dee U. Silverthorn, *Human Physiology: An Integrated Approach*, 4th ed. (San Francisco, CA: Pearson Education, Inc, 2009), p. 458.
[51]Ellen G. White, *Christ Triumphant* (Hagerstown, MD: Review and Herald, 1999), p. 20.
[52]Ellen G. White, *Education* (Mountain View, CA: Pacific Press, 1903), p. 215.
[53]"The 4 Components of a good exercise programme," health24, https://1ref.us/1ey (accessed May 11, 2020).
[54]Edward R. Laskowski, "How much should the average adult exercise every day?" Mayo Clinic, https://1ref.us/1ez (accessed May 11, 2020).
[55]Gina D. Wagner, "Strength in Numbers: The Importance of Fitness Buddies," 2Unstoppable, https://1ref.us/1f0 (accessed May 11, 2020).

Spiritually speaking, there is a need for us to exercise our faith in God. While physically, walking may be the best exercise activity, the Bible talks about running with perseverance the race marked out for us:

> Therefore, since we are surrounded by such a great cloud of witnesses, let us throw off everything that hinders and the sin that so easily entangles. And let us run with perseverance the race marked out for us, fixing our eyes on Jesus, the pioneer and perfecter of faith. For the joy set before him he endured the cross, scorning its shame, and sat down at the right hand of the throne of God. Consider him who endured such opposition from sinners, so that you will not grow weary and lose heart. (Heb. 12:1–3, NIV)

Our run of faith is more like a marathon, where what is important is not being the first to the finish line but finishing the run all the way to the end. Consider what the apostle Paul counsels us about the discipline needed to finish the marathon of faith:

> Do you not know that in a race all the runners run, but only one receives the prize? So run that you may obtain it. Every athlete exercises self-control in all things. They do it to receive a perishable wreath, but we an imperishable. So, I do not run aimlessly; I do not box as one beating the air. But I discipline my body and keep it under control, lest after preaching to others I myself should be disqualified. (1 Cor. 9:24–27, ESV)

"So be careful how you live. Don't live like fools, but like those who are wise. Make the most of every opportunity in these evil days" (Eph. 5:15–16, NLT).

Wholistic exercise is conducive to radical wellness in accordance with how God designed us to live. If you want to experience radical wellness, as Nike's slogan says, "Just do it." Exercise your mind, body and spirit—to the glory of God and the blessing of yourself, your family and your fellow men.

Our run of faith is more like a marathon, where what is important is not being the first to the finish line but finishing the run all the way to the end.

Benefits of exercise. Here are some of the benefits of physical activity:

"By active exercise in the open air every day, the liver, kidneys, and lungs also will be strengthened to perform their work."[56]

Physical activities have corollary benefits to the mind: "Work of brain and muscle is beneficial. Each faculty of the mind and each muscle of the body has its distinctive office, and all require exercise to develop them and give them healthful vigor. Each wheel in the living mechanism must be brought into use. The whole organism needs to be constantly exercised in order to be efficient and meet the object of its creation."[57]

"Since the mind and the soul find expression through the body, both mental and spiritual vigor are in great degree dependent upon physical strength and activity; whatever promotes physical health promotes the development of a strong mind and a well-balanced character."[58] Exercise reverses effects of prolonged stress on the anatomy and physiology of the brain.[59]

Beneficial whole-person activities. Since a human being is not only a body, it goes that one can also reap the benefits from mental and spiritual exercises:

"The truths of the Bible, received, will uplift mind and soul. If the Word of God were appreciated as it should be, both young and old would possess an inward rectitude, a strength of principle, that would enable them to resist temptation."[60]

There are great, whole-person benefits from worshipping and praising God: "It is good to give thanks to the LORD, to sing praises to the Most High. It is good to proclaim your unfailing love in the morning, your faithfulness in the evening" (Ps. 92:1–2, NLT).

As co-workers with God, we are mandated to exercise our spirituality by participating in working out God's plan and purposes on planet earth. "[We] must work the works of him that sent [us] … while it is day: the night cometh, when no man can work" (John 9:4, KJV).

Great beneficial results await those who work with God in the salvation of people in the world. We see this truth from the experience of Jesus Christ and His disciples' ministry to the Samaritans, as recorded in the

[56]Ellen G. White, *Counsels on Health* (Mountain View, CA: Pacific Press, 1923), p. 54.
[57]Ellen G. White, *Christ Triumphant* (Hagerstown, MD: Review and Herald, 1999), p. 20.
[58]Ellen G. White, *Mind, Character, and Personality*, vol. 2 (Hagerstown, MD: Review and Herald, 1977), p. 406.
[59]Suptendra N. Sarbadhikari and Asit K. Saha, "Moderate exercise and chronic stress produce counteractive effects on different areas of the brain by acting through various neurotransmitter receptor subtypes: A hypothesis," National Center for Biotechnology Information, https://1ref.us/1f1 (accessed May 11, 2020).
[60]Ellen G. White, *Mind, Character, and Personality*, vol. 1 (Hagerstown, MD: Review and Herald, 1977), p. 89.

Bible: "You may say that there are still four months until harvest time. But I tell you to look, and you will see that the fields are ripe and ready to harvest …. A lot of Samaritans in that town put their faith in Jesus because [of what] the woman had said … [and] [m]any more Samaritans put their faith in Jesus because of what they heard him say" (John 4:35, 39, 41, CEV).

The need for adequate rest. A person needs to engage in regular physical exercise as well as have adequate and periodic rest. Even the most active organ of the body (the heart) must rest between heartbeats.

Exercising, relaxing and getting enough rest will help you do better and enjoy life more. Getting the correct amount of quality sleep is essential to your ability to learn and process memories. Additionally, sleep helps restore your body's energy, repair muscle tissue and triggers the release of hormones that affect growth and appetite.[61]

In the beginning, God provided the seventh-day Sabbath as a regular period of physical rest for man:

> Remember the sabbath day, to keep it holy. Six days shalt thou labour, and do all thy work: But the seventh day is the sabbath of the LORD thy God: in it thou shalt not do any work, thou, nor thy son, nor thy daughter, thy manservant, nor thy maidservant, nor thy cattle, nor thy stranger that is within thy gates: For in six days the LORD made heaven and earth, the sea, and all that in them is, and rested the seventh day: wherefore the LORD blessed the sabbath day, and hallowed it. (Exod. 20:8–11, KJV)

As for our need for spiritual rest, Jesus Christ said: "Come unto me, all ye that labour and are heavy laden, and I will give you rest. Take my yoke upon you, and learn of me; for I am meek and lowly in heart: and ye shall find rest unto your souls. For my yoke is easy, and my burden is light" (Matt. 11:28–30, KJV).

---

[61]"Four crucial ways that sleep helps the body to heal," *Chicago Tribune*, https://1ref.us/1f2 (accessed July 9, 2020).

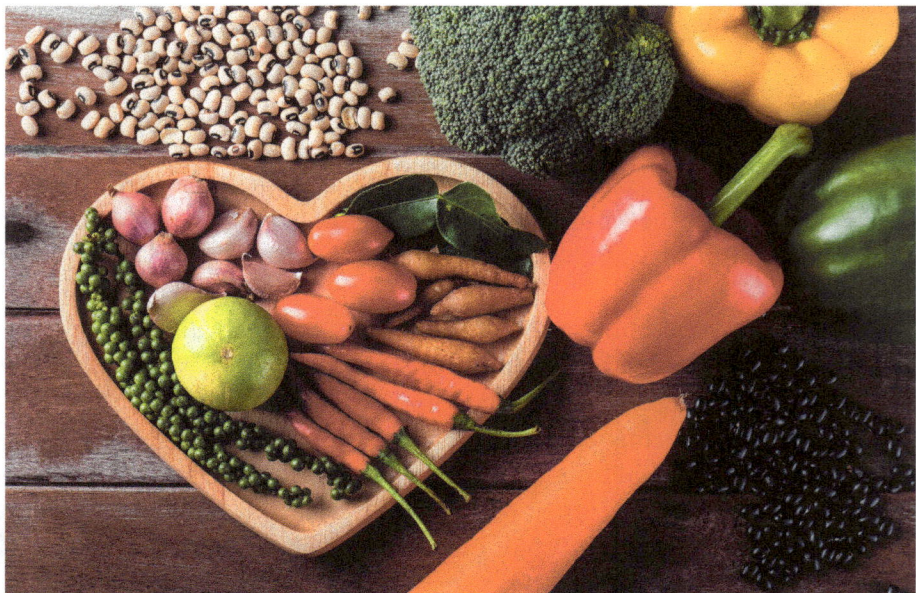

Chapter 6

Eat Designer Foods—They're the Best for You

Blessed Wellness Habit Number 6

"D iet is the essential key to all successful healing."[62]
There is no question about the relationship between nutrition and wellness. Wellness experts say that nutrition is the anchor for meaningful living. In fact, nutrition and wellness have become quite synonymous, especially with the advent of aggressive advertising of so-called wellness companies promoting their nutritional supplements. In this chapter, we shall discuss five key principles in eating right: the right kind, variety, amount, time to eat and motive.

---

[62]Joseph R. Raymond, "Nutrition Sayings and Quotes," Wise Old Sayings, https://1ref.us/1f3 (accessed May 11, 2020).

The right kind of food. The American College of Lifestyle Medicine (ACLM) recommends good food as one way to boost the immune system: "Healthy Eating. What you eat makes all the difference! For strong immunity, consume a wide array of fiber-filled, nutrient-dense, and antioxidant-rich whole plant foods at every meal. Choose a rainbow of fruits and vegetables, eat your beans, consume whole grains, and use a variety of herbs and spices to enhance flavors. Stay hydrated with water!"[63]

Groundbreaking research such as *The China Study*, Adventist Health Study I and II, among many others, has established the causal relationship between healthy eating habits and good health.

Actually, the choice that ACLM recommends—to "consume a wide array of fiber-filled, nutrient-dense, and anti-oxidant-rich whole plant foods at every meal"[64]—is basic Bible stuff. That is the menu that our Creator God designed and gave man for food.

In the beginning, God provided the best nutritional resources for man. "He who created man and who understands his needs appointed Adam his food. 'Behold,' He said, 'I have given you every herb yielding seed, … and every tree, in which is the fruit of a tree yielding seed; to you it shall be for food.' Upon leaving Eden to gain his livelihood by tilling the earth under the curse of sin, man received permission to eat also 'the herb of the field.'"[65]

Scientific nutrition research evidence agrees with the above: "Healthy eating may be best achieved with a plant-based diet, which we define as a regimen that encourages whole, plant-based foods and

> *What you eat makes all the difference! For strong immunity, consume a wide array of fiber-filled, nutrient-dense, and antioxidant-rich whole plant foods at every meal. Choose a rainbow of fruits and vegetables, eat your beans, consume whole grains, and use a variety of herbs and spices to enhance flavors. Stay hydrated with water!"*

[63]"Lifestyle Choices to Boost immunity," American College of Lifestyle Medicine, https://1ref.us/1f4 (accessed May 11, 2020).
[64]"Lifestyle Choices."
[65]Ellen G. White, *Counsels on Diet and Foods* (Washington, DC: Review and Herald, 1938), p. 81.

discourages meats, dairy products, and eggs as well as all refined and processed foods."[66]

Hans Diehl, DHSc, popularized the term "foods-as-grown."[67] That is the kind of diet he recommended in the well-known and successful Complete Health Improvement Program (CHIP), which he founded.[68]

Some health educators suggest that human beings were designed to be vegetarians. They argue that the human teeth anatomy is not designed for eating meat.[69]

Dietary research evidence suggests the advantages of a plant-based diet. Researchers tracked 73,309 Adventists who followed the church's dietary counsel of plant-based diet to varying degrees. The study showed that vegetarians experienced 12 percent fewer deaths over a six-year period of research.[70]

Sylvester Graham, a Presbyterian minister and dietary reformer in the middle of the nineteenth century promoted eating only raw foods as a way to avoid illness.[71]

A raw vegan diet focusing on fruits, vegetables, nuts, seeds, sprouted whole grains and legumes may improve overall health. This kind of diet has been consistently linked to lower blood pressures and a reduced risk of heart disease and stroke.

"Observational studies report that vegans may have up to a 75% lower risk of developing high blood pressure and a 42% lower risk of dying from heart disease. What's more, several randomized controlled studies—the gold standard in scientific research—observe that vegan diets are particularly effective at reducing 'bad' LDL cholesterol."[72]

My wife Beth and I usually attend lectures (especially if they are free) on topics related to our Radical Wellness advocacy. Recently we attended one given by a nutritionist at the local health education center of our healthcare provider group. The lecturer summarized what comprises a

---

[66]Philip Tuso, Mohamed Ismail, Benjamin Ha, and Carole Bartolotto, "Nutritional Update for Physicians: Plant-Based Diets," National Center for Biotechnology Information, https://1ref.us/1f5 (accessed May 11, 2020).

[67]"Live More," Lifestyle Medicine Institute, https://1ref.us/1f6 (accessed July 9, 2020).

[68]"Complete Health Improvement Program," Lifestyle Medicine Institute, https://1ref.us/1fu (accessed November 5, 2020).

[69]Barbara King, "Humans are 'Meathooked' But Not Designed For Meat-Eating," National Public Radio, https://1ref.us/1f7 (accessed May 11, 2020).

[70]"Vegetarian Diets Associated With Lower Risk of Death," JAMA Network, https://1ref.us/1f8 (accessed May 11, 2020).

[71]Alina Petre, "How to Follow a Raw Vegan Diet: Benefits and Risks," healthline, https://1ref.us/1f9 (accessed July 9, 2020).

[72]Petre, "Raw Vegan."

healthy personal dietary practice by giving us two simple acronyms: *CCC* and *SOS.*

In order to ensure that we are getting good food, she said that we should avoid ingesting what are *C*rispy, *C*heesy and *C*reamy foods. She added that when we go shopping, we should be on the lookout for and avoid grabbing products from the grocery shelves that are awash in *S*alt, *O*il and *S*ugar. She taught us how to read and understand those cryptic food labels on canned and packaged food products.

The right variety. "Grains, fruits, nuts, and vegetables constitute the diet chosen for us by our Creator. These foods, prepared in as simple and natural a manner as possible, are the most healthful and nourishing. They impart a strength, a power of endurance, and a vigor of intellect, that are not afforded by a more complex and stimulating diet."[73]

After the flood, man began eating a meat diet. The Bible delineates the variety of clean and unclean meat.

> God created two basic classes of animals in relation to man's diet. Those that benefit our health are called clean foods and those that do not (they are a detriment to our health and well being) are labeled in the Bible as unclean. We find this critical information regarding which meats are good for us (clean) and which are not (unclean) in Leviticus 11 and Deuteronomy 14.
>
> In spite of what many believers think, the Bible does not, in the Old or New Testaments, abolish or do away with God's laws about foods that he created either to be eaten (clean) or avoided (unclean).[74]

The benefits and blessing of eating Bible-delineated clean food was showcased in the experience of Daniel and his friends who refused to eat what was served in the King of Babylon's food court.

> Daniel decided not to eat the king's food and wine because that would make him unclean …. Daniel said to the guard, "Please give us this test for ten days: Don't give us anything but vegetables to eat and water to drink …. So, the guard agreed to test them for ten days. After ten days they looked very healthy. They looked better than all of the young men who ate the king's food. So, the guard

[73]Ellen G. White, *Counsels on Diet and Foods* (Washington, DC: Review and Herald, 1938), p. 81.
[74]"What are clean and unclean foods?" Bible Study, https://1ref.us/1fa (accessed May 11, 2020).

took away the king's special food and wine … [feeding them] vegetables instead. (Dan. 1:8, 12, 14–16, ICB)

What was the result of Daniel and his friends' strict adherence to biblically prescribed food?

At the end of the time, when the king had commanded that they should be brought in, the chief of the eunuchs brought them in before Nebuchadnezzar. And the king spoke with them, and among all of them none was found like Daniel, Hananiah, Mishael, and Azariah. Therefore they stood before the king. And in every matter of wisdom and understanding about which the king inquired of them, he found them ten times better than all the magicians and enchanters that were in all his kingdom. (Dan. 1:18–20, ESV)

Even foods that are good may not be suitable to eat, depending on the situation:

But not all foods wholesome in themselves are equally suited to our needs under all circumstances. Care should be taken in the selection of food. Our diet should be suited to the season, to the climate in which we live, and to the occupation we follow. Some foods that are adapted for use at one season or in one climate are not suited to another. Likewise, there are different foods best suited for persons in different occupations. Often food that can be used with benefit by those engaged in hard physical labor is unsuitable for persons of sedentary pursuits or intense mental application. God has given us an ample variety of healthful foods, and we should choose from it the things that experience and sound judgment prove to be best suited to our own individual necessities.[75]

The right amount. Judicious eating habits are crucial to radical wellness. Even good food becomes harmful if too much is eaten. There is need for self-control in eating.

Many are suffering, and many are going into the grave, because of the indulgence of appetite. They eat what suits their perverted taste, thus weakening the digestive organs and injuring their power to assimilate the food that is to sustain life. This brings on acute

---

[75]Ellen G. White, *The Ministry of Healing* (Mountain View, CA: Pacific Press, 1905), pp. 296–297.

disease, and too often death follows. The delicate organism of the body is worn out by the suicidal practices of those who ought to know better.[76]

"The system receives less nourishment from too great a quantity of food, even of the right quality, than from a moderate quantity taken at regular periods."[77]

Here is one practical example of the wisdom of temperate eating. A newspaper in Singapore reported a study on eating rice. The report stated that "each plate of white rice eaten in a day—on a regular basis—raises the risk of diabetes by 11 per cent in the overall population."[78]

The right time. Some people regularly eat three times a day; some only two times. Here are the recommended times for eating three regular meals a day:

You should eat within the first hour of waking to get your body primed for a successful day. Between 6 and 10 a.m. would be the ideal time to take this first meal, mainly so that you set yourself up for a second meal a few hours later ....

Your metabolism peaks each day between 10 a.m. and 2 p.m. Aim to eat lunch between these hours to take advantage of stronger digestive function at this time ....

You should eat dinner approximately four to five hours after eating lunch. If that falls in the 5 p.m. to 6 p.m. window, you hit the last hour of your body's heightened metabolic rate before it starts to slow.[79]

Dinner should not be eaten late at night. The practice of late-night eating raises the risk of coronary heart disease. "Compared with men who did not eat late at night, those who ate late at night had a 55% higher CHD risk."[80]

[76]Ellen G. White, *Counsels on Diet and Foods* (Washington, DC: Review and Herald, 1938), p. 123.
[77]White, *Diet and Foods*, p. 103.
[78]"Diabetes: The rice you eat is worse than sugary drinks," *The Straits Times*, https://1ref.us/1fb (accessed May 11, 2020).
[79]"WHEN IS THE BEST TIME TO EAT BREAKFAST, LUNCH, AND DINNER?" Forklift and Palate, https://1ref.us/1fc (accessed May 11, 2020).
[80]Leah Cahill, Stephanie Chiuve, Rania Mekary, Majken Jensen, Alan Flint, Frank Hu and Eric Rimm, "A Prospective Study of Breakfast Eating and Incident Coronary Heart Disease in a Cohort of Male U.S. Health Professionals," National Center for Biotechnology Information, https://1ref.us/1fd (accessed May 11, 2020).

The right motive. For those people who like to honor God, eating can be done in such a way as to glorify Him. They believe that the "body is the temple of the Holy Spirit" (1 Cor. 6:19). Since they believe that their body is the temple of the Holy Spirit, they eat the right kind, variety and amount of food at the right time with the right motive.

One of the cardinal lessons I learned from my health classes both in college and graduate school was that eating can be a form of worship. I remember a Bible verse that definitely suggests that concept: "So, whether you eat or drink, or whatever you do, do all to the glory of God" (1 Cor. 10:31, ESV).

As for the best mental and spiritual diet, consider this story: One day, one of my instructors in vocational nursing school told a story of a missionary family who lived and served somewhere in the jungles of South America. With exposure to a new environment, all three of the missionary couples' young daughters tragically soon died. Distraught and depressed, the man wandered aimlessly, unaware of his surroundings.

Soon he found himself in a gathering; a séance was going on. As he walked toward the front of the meeting place, his three dead daughters suddenly appeared, running towards him. His immediate reflex was to scoop them up with his arms.

In short, the missionary man found himself before the medium. Curious, he asked the devil through the medium what he, the devil, would do to deceive the world into believing his lies about God. The devil replied that he would tell him his secret weapon of deception on the condition that he would not reveal his answer to any other person, or else he would die.

Apparently, we know what happened to the missionary because we now know what the devil's answer to his question was—his method of deceiving the whole world was disseminating lies about God through the "idiot box." The story happened many years ago, according to my nursing instructor. As we now know, the media can be a very effective medium of spiritual deception. On the other hand, God's Word—the Bible—speaks the truth about God and how we may be saved from the devil's delusions and eternal destruction.

"The Bible contains all the principles that men need to understand in order to be fitted either for this life or for the life to come. And these principles may be understood by all."[81]

---

[81]Ellen G. White, *Education* (Mountain View, CA: Pacific Press, 1903), p. 123.

For our overall health, consider this recommendation for the best mental and spiritual diet from the Bible: "Finally brothers and sisters, whatever is true, whatever is honorable, whatever is just, whatever is pure, whatever is lovely, whatever is commendable—if there is any moral excellence and if there is anything praiseworthy—dwell on these things" (Phil. 4:8, CSB).

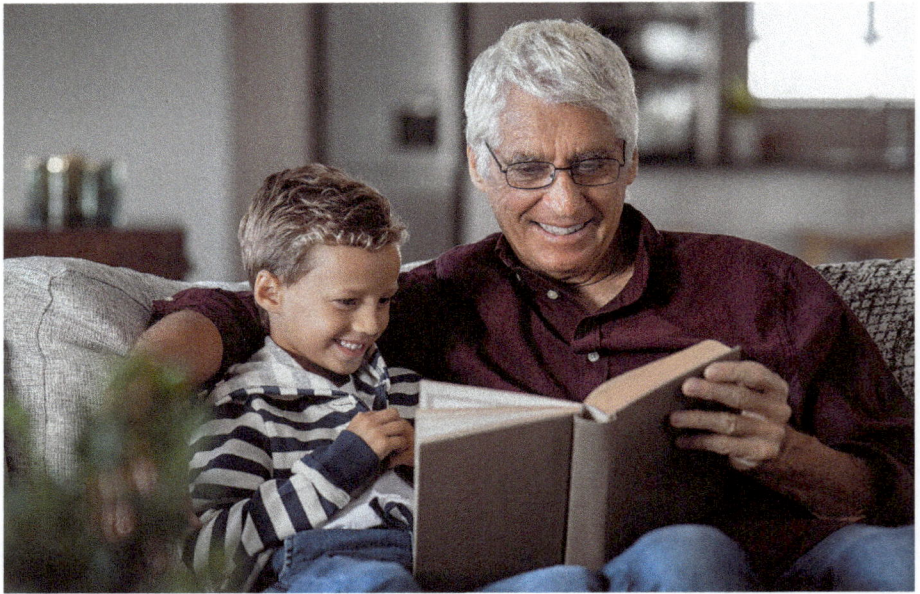

Chapter 7

Live Vibrantly with Purpose and Hope

Blessed Wellness Habit Number 7

D id you know that if you did all the seven blessed habits to radical wellness, you will still die when your time comes?

However long you live in this dispensation, the Bible says, "For everything there is a season, and a time for every matter under heaven: a time to be born, and a time to die" (Eccles. 3:1–2, ESV).

Consider the life span of men from Eden to the great flood: From Adam to Enoch, the average life span was 838 years. In these seven generations, the longest lived was Jared (960 years) and the shortest lived was Enoch (365 years). The Bible says that Enoch is still alive today. God took him to heaven because he "walked with God" (Gen. 5:24, ESV).

From Methuselah (Enoch's son) to Noah (the last patriarch before the flood)—three generations—the average life span was 899 years. So, the total average life span of men before the flood was 869 years. After the flood, the average life span of men (from Arphaxad to King David) dramatically plummeted to 253 years.[82] By the time of King David, "the days of … [man's] years … [were just] threescore years and ten [70]; and if by reason of strength they be fourscore years [80], yet is their strength labour and sorrow; for it is soon cut off, and … [they] fly away" (Ps. 90:10, KJV).

In 2017, the average American lived 78.6 years, according to the report from the National Center for Health Statistics.[83] Worldwide, the "United Nations estimate a global average life expectancy of 72.6 years for 2019."[84]

In the beginning. When God created man, He intended that he live forever. God created man in His image. "So God created man in His *own* image; in the image of God He created him; male and female He created them" (Gen. 1:27).

When God created man, He created him with a capacity for never-ending development. "God created man in his own image" (Genesis 1:27), and it was His purpose that the longer man lived the more fully he should reveal this image—the more fully reflect the glory of the Creator. All his faculties were capable of development; their capacity and vigor were continually to increase."[85]

Neuroscience has recently discovered that indeed man has the capability for never-ending development. The human brain has this characteristic called neuroplasticity; it is built to last for eternity. "Neuroplasticity refers to the lifelong capacity of the brain to change and rewire itself in response to the stimulation of learning and experience. Neurogenesis is the ability to create new neurons and connections between neurons throughout a lifetime."[86]

So, why do people die? The Bible's answer is straightforward and direct. People die because of sin: "For the wages of sin *is* death" (Rom. 6:23). "[F]or all have sinned and fall short of the glory of God" (Rom. 3:23, NIV).

---

[82]"How old were the Biblical patriarchs?" Bible Study, https://1ref.us/1fe (accessed April 15, 2020).

[83]Laura Santhanam, "American life expectancy has dropped again. Here's why," PBS News Hour, https://1ref.us/1ff (accessed April 15, 2020).

[84]Max Roser, Esteban Ortiz-Ospina and Hannah Ritchie, "Life Expectancy," Our World in Data, https://1ref.us/1fg (accessed April 15, 2020).

[85]Ellen G. White, *Reflecting Christ* (Hagerstown, MD: Review and Herald, 2008), p. 105.

[86]Alvaro Fernandez, Elkhonon Goldberg, and Pascale Michelon, "Neuroplasticity: the potential for lifelong brain development," Sharp Brains, https://1ref.us/1fh (accessed April 15, 2020).

When God created Adam and Eve in His image, He gave them the freedom of choice; they were free to obey Him willingly or they could disobey Him. Their continued existence was predicated on their continued obedience to God. God loved them so much and desired that they develop a character of continued trust and obedience. He gave them a provision in Eden for that opportunity. "And the LORD God commanded him, 'You may eat freely from every tree of the garden, but you must not eat from the tree of the knowledge of good and evil; for in the day that you eat of it, you will surely die'" (Gen. 2:16–17, BSB).

When Adam and Eve made a wrong choice, they were banished from Eden. They should have died the moment they sinned but the blood of "the Lamb ... slain from the foundation of the world" (Rev. 13:8) shielded them and the whole world from instant and eternal destruction.

Instead of disappearing into oblivion, they and their descendants were given a second chance in Jesus Christ. He came to earth as the Savior so that sinners like you and I can have eternal life. "The Word became flesh and made his dwelling among us. We have seen his glory, the glory of the one and only Son, who came from the Father, full of grace and truth. Out of his fullness we have all received grace in place of grace already given" (John 1:14, 16, NIV).

So, that is where we are still today. Every one of us will die the natural death because we are all sinners. "For the wages of sin is death [but there is a way of escape from eternal death because], ... the free gift of God is eternal life through Christ Jesus our Lord" (Rom. 6:23, NLT).

The fine-tuned universe. God could not just say to us "I forgive you" and forego the consequence of our sin. That is because of the nature of the universe that He created. It is so fine-tuned that a moral disobedience threatens it with physical disaster.

> The same power that upholds nature, is working also in man. The same great laws that guide alike the star and the atom control human life. The laws that govern the heart's action, regulating the flow of the current of life to the body, are the laws of the mighty Intelligence that has the jurisdiction of the soul. From Him all life proceeds. Only in harmony with Him can be found its true sphere of action. For all the objects of His creation the condition is the same—a life sustained by receiving the life of God, a life exercised in harmony with the Creator's will. To transgress His law, physical,

mental, or moral, is to place one's self out of harmony with the universe, to introduce discord, anarchy, ruin.[87]

It took the death of the Creator of the universe, Jesus Christ, to bridge the gap between God and man because of sin. Jesus Christ had to be incarnated, live a perfect life of obedience to God and die, though without sin, to restore humanity to the original harmony and unity with divinity.

The Bible explains God's amazing love gift to sinners thus: "Therefore, as by the offence of one [Adam] judgment came upon all men to condemnation; even so by the righteousness of one [Jesus Christ] the free gift came upon all men unto justification of life. For as by one man's disobedience many were made sinners, so by the obedience of one shall many be made righteous" (Rom. 5:18–19, KJV).

The pale blue dot.

It took the death of the Creator of the universe, Jesus Christ, to bridge the gap between God and man because of sin. Jesus Christ had to be incarnated, live a perfect life of obedience to God and die, though without sin, to restore humanity to the original harmony and unity with divinity.

The Pale Blue Dot is a photograph of planet Earth taken on February 14, 1990, by the *Voyager 1* space probe from a record distance of about 6 billion kilometers (3.7 billion miles, 40.5 AU), as part of that day's *Family Portrait* series of images of the Solar System.

In the photograph, Earth's apparent size is less than a pixel; the planet appears as a tiny dot against the vastness of space, among bands of sunlight reflected by the camera.[88]

I cited this fact here because, to me, it shows an amazing perspective of the indescribable love of God for sinners like you and me. Reflecting on that amazing picture, the late celebrated astronomer Carl Sagan described earth as a mere "mote of dust suspended in a sunbeam."[89] When man sinned, God could have just extinguished that insignificant, rebellious

[87]Ellen G. White, *Education* (Mountain View, CA: Pacific Press, 1903), pp. 99–100.
[88]"*Pale Blue Dot*," Wikipedia, https://1ref.us/1fi (accessed April 15, 2020).
[89]Carol Sagan, "A Pale Blue Dot," The Planetary Society, https://1ref.us/1fj (accessed April 15, 2020).

"mote of dust" into oblivion. But His amazing love couldn't and wouldn't let Him do it. "For God so loved the world, that he gave his only begotten Son, that whosoever believeth in him should not perish, but have everlasting life" (John 3:16, KJV).

I love that word "whosoever" because it includes the name of one sinner, Libni A. Cerdenio, in there—and billions of other names too.

❋❋❋❋

Let me just share with you one personal experience on how God makes a way to show His love to even just one person who needs to know about it. I like to tell this story as "The Texas-Romania-Switzerland Connection:"

In April 1997, I joined a Quiet Hour evangelistic team to hold health and gospel outreach meetings in Romania. Our memorable three-week stint in the small, ancient city of Dej, close to the Ukrainian border, was over. After the baptism of twenty-one new believers on a symbolic day when the whole countryside was covered with snow, our host drove us overnight over the mountainous Transylvania terrain to Bucharest where we were to board our flight back to the USA. When we reached the airport, I was aghast to learn that while my two friends were boarding the plane in a few hours on a straight flight to California, I was going to spend that day and night in Bucharest. The following day, I would board a connecting flight to Zurich, and lay over there for another night! I was too dismayed to even question our host—who arranged our homeward itinerary—why in the world that had happened to me.

So, as my two friends were eagerly anticipating a safe landing at LAX after a sixteen-hour flight with a brief stopover in Amsterdam, I was perfunctorily on a tour through Bucharest and an overnight stay in my host's spartan apartment in the heart of the city.

When I landed in Zurich the next evening, a pastor-friend of our Romanian host met me at the airport. He whisked me straight to the midweek prayer meeting of some German-speaking believers in his church. He requested me to speak to the small group. First, I gave them a brief report of our meetings in Dej, Romania. I was then inspired to share with them the reality of God's existence as proven by His special revelation to me during a time of personal struggle when I was a new immigrant in the small city of Pecos, in the southwest of the vast state of Texas.

I related to them how one day God answered my simple, childlike prayer while I was going to vocational nursing school at the Winkler

County Memorial Hospital in Kermit, Texas. (If you remember, I told this story in Chapter 1).

When the church pastor was driving us home through the narrow, winding city roads of Zurich, he intimated to me what one old lady in the small group at church told him after the service.

The elderly widow lived under communist Romania for many years. In that kind of life, it was quite hard for her to believe in God. But my testimony so moved her that she could now believe in the existence of a loving, benevolent God.

Looking back, I praise God for that providentially delayed itinerary back home so one elderly person in Zurich could see a glimpse of God's amazing love!

❖❖❖❖

How to live forever. The Bible says, "There is salvation in no one else, for there is no other name under heaven given among mortals by which we must be saved" (Acts 4:12, NRSV).

My friend, the health and wellness continuum extend forever and ever in the earth made new. Salvation in Jesus Christ is the restoration and eternal perpetuation of life, health and happiness.

How amazing, wonderful, and gracious is God's love for you and me! If we accept Jesus Christ as Savior and the Lord of our life, we can live vibrantly with purpose and hope today.

In heaven, we will enjoy perfect health forever and ever!

My friend, the health and wellness continuum extend forever and ever in the earth made new. Salvation in Jesus Christ is the restoration and eternal perpetuation of life, health and happiness.

Conclusion

Accept the Giver, Receive the Gift

The experience of Nicolaus Copernicus in discovering that the earth revolves around the sun and not otherwise, is evidence that there are immutable realities we can discover if we do away with traditional perceptions and embrace that which we find out by careful study and investigation.

That is what I have attempted to convey in *Seven Blessed Habits to Radical Wellness*. At the outset, I proposed that radical health and wellness is not a status that we need to work for or attain, rather it is a gift that we have to accept from God.

The Bible says, "Whatever is good and perfect is a gift coming down to us from God our Father .... He never changes or casts a shifting shadow" (James 1:17, NLT).

As I was writing this book, I could see the slowly but surely rising steel main frame of the new seventeen-story building of the Loma Linda University Medical Center and Children's Hospital above the fruit-tree-lined horizon beyond our backyard. I saw the daily progress of this building construction. I saw how deep into the ground the foundation was set.

Dig deep to build high is a principle that is applicable in building our house of health. Building on the foundational principles of life, health and happiness found in the Bible—the Creator's revealed will for human life—will ensure success in our quest for eternal health and wellness.

Jesus Christ told a parable which is most relevant to this subject. He said:

> Anyone who listens to my teaching and follows it is wise, like a person who builds a house on solid rock. Though the rain comes in torrents and the floodwaters rise and the winds beat against that house, it won't collapse because it is built on bedrock. But anyone who hears my teaching and doesn't obey it is foolish, like a person who builds a house on sand. When the rains and floods come and the winds beat against that house, it will collapse with a mighty crash. (Matt. 7:24–27, NLT)

Building the house of health is an adjunct method that we at Wellness Plus Institute teach. God is the *bedrock* on which a healthy and happy life can be built. Our choices to embrace God's provisions for us to not only exist but to thrive is the stable *foundation* on which we build. The atmosphere, healthy relationships, exercise or adequate physical activity and rest and nutrition are the *pillars* that support a life of optimal health. All of these elements are covered in place by the *roof* of God's salvation. Because of His love, God created us and planned and put into effect the process of saving us from the consequences of our individual and collective wrong choices—diseases, temporal and eternal death. The *walls* of the house of health represent our obedience to God's physical and spiritual health laws. Grateful obedience as a response to His saving and sanctifying love ensures the blessings of temporal and eternal health and happiness.

Matthew the Gospel writer narrated Jesus Christ's parable of building on the Rock. It is in the context of Him teaching the multitude on a mountain (Matt. 5:1). His long discourse begins in Matthew 5.

Before He told the people this story, Jesus told the people about hypocrisy (Matt. 7:1–6), saying that His followers should not be judgmental, but rather focus on their own need for improvement and redemption.

He then gave them a lovely picture of God who desires to grant our desires to be and do good. He said that heaven's resources to grant our desires for goodness are unlimited (Matt. 7:7–12). Jesus said that we should keep asking, seeking and knocking at heaven's door because God is more than willing to give good things to them who ask Him (verse 11). As one enlightened writer said: "All His biddings are enablings."[90]

Further, Jesus Christ said that building a life of faith and faithfulness requires stringent discipline or obedience to God's physical and moral health laws. It is like entering a narrow gate which "leads to life" (verse 14).

Then Jesus said that men should beware of following false prophets or teachers who profess to help you but are subtly trying to help themselves. They come not to guide you to life but to your eternal destruction (verses 15–20). The way to see who they really are is through their fruits (verse 20). This brings me to my belief that Ellen G. White was a true prophet.[91] Look at the magnitude of her influence seen in people, schools and hospitals all over the world!

Jesus Christ warned the people about false prophets and teachers because many who profess to know and follow Him are not and don't do His will (verses 21–23).

There are two classes of people who profess to know and follow Christ. They are represented in His story of the wise and foolish men building their houses on the rock and sand, respectively. He spoke about who are His real and false followers. Many will profess and declare themselves to be followers of Christ, but He said He does not know them (Matt. 7:23).

Let me share with you a paragraph that I read about the meaning of the parable of the wise and foolish men: "The spiritual meaning of the parable is found in Matthew 7:24: 'Everyone who hears these words of mine and puts them into practice is like a wise man who built his house on the rock.' We are each building a life. The proper foundation for a life is Jesus' words—not just the hearing … [of them, but the doing of them too (see James 1:22)]."[92]

Before I close this conclusion to the *Seven Blessed Habits to Radical Wellness*, I would like to propose that the parable about the wise and foolish men is about living a life of health, wellness, happiness and joy.

Immediately after Jesus taught the people about this parable, He went down the mountain and healed a leper (Matt. 8:1–4), the Centurion's sick

---

[90]Ellen G. White, *Christ's Object Lessons* (Mountain View, CA: Pacific Press, 1900), p. 333.

[91]Theodore Levterov, "A True Prophet …" Adventist, https://1ref.us/1fk (accessed May 7, 2020).

[92]"What does it mean that the wise man built his house upon a rock?" Got Questions, https://1ref. us/1fv (accessed November 5, 2020).

servant (Matt. 8:5–13), Peter's mother-in-law (Matt. 8:14–15) and many more (Matt. 8:16–17).

My dear friends, if we accept Jesus Christ into our lives, we receive God's gift of radical wellness. For He "came that … [we] may have life and have it abundantly" (John 10:10, ESV).

The hymn "Trust and Obey" expresses the eternal truth that obedience and gratitude to God for His gifts is the solid ground on which we can truly build a life of real health and wellness:

TRUST AND OBEY
When we walk with the Lord in the light of His word,
What a glory He sheds on our way!
While we do His good will, He abides with us still,
And with all who will trust and obey.

Refrain
Trust and obey, for there's no other way
To be happy in Jesus, but to trust and obey.

Not a burden we bear, Not a sorrow we share,
But our toil he doth richly repay;
Not a grief nor a loss, Not a frown nor a cross,
But is blest if we trust and obey. [Refrain]

But we never can prove The delights of His love,
Until all on the altar we lay,
For the favor He shows, And the joy He bestows,
Are for them who will trust and obey. [Refrain]

Then in fellowship sweet We will sit at His feet,
Or we'll walk by His side in the way;
What He says we will do, Where He sends we will go,
Never fear, only trust and obey. [Refrain][93]

---

[93]John H. Sammis, "Trust and Obey," *Seventh-day Adventist Hymnal*, Review and Herald, 1985.

About the Author

L ibni A. Cerdenio is a former Associate Editor of Philippine Publishing House where he edited *Health & Home*, the Philippines' *National Journal of Better Living*. He has a graduate theology degree from the SDA Theological Seminary (Far East), now Adventist International Institute of Advanced Studies (AIIAS). He is licensed as a registered nurse (RN) in the state of California, USA.

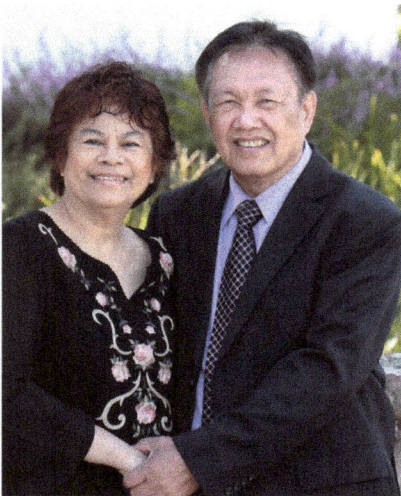

He and his wife Elizabeth (née Timbancaya-Mingua) are the founders of Wellness Plus Institute, a wholistic health teaching ministry which they do as an extension of their professional role as registered nurses and a fulfillment of their civic duty as citizens of the world. They do social media "radical wellness" evangelism. They have conducted GARDENS (a theocentric and gospel-oriented model of health promotion and education) seminars in church and non-church venues, both in the USA and in the Philippines.

Libni A. Cerdenio is a member of the American College of Lifestyle Medicine (ACLM).

Bibliography

Bates, Todd. "What will it take to live on the moon?" Phys.org. https://1ref. us/1ei (accessed May 5, 2020).

"How old were the Biblical patriarchs?" Bible Study. https://1ref.us/1fe (accessed April 15, 2020).

Brady, David. "Health Benefits of Grounding (Earthing)." The Fibro Fix. https://1ref.us/1ep (accessed May 11, 2020).

Burch, Kelly. "Loneliness may weaken the immune system — here's how to feel less lonely during social isolation." Insider. https://1ref.us/1et (accessed May 11, 2020).

Cahill, Leah, Stephanie Chiuve, Rania Mekary, Majken Jensen, Alan Flint, Frank Hu, and Eric Rimm. "A Prospective Study of Breakfast Eating and Incident Coronary Heart Disease in a Cohort of Male U.S. Health Professionals." National Center for Biotechnology Information. https://1ref.us/1fd (accessed May 11, 2020).

Chopra, D., and R. Tanzi. *The Healing Self: A Revolutionary New Plan to Supercharge Your Immunity and Stay Well for Life.* New York, NY: Harmony Books, 2018.

Clear, James. "The Physics of Productivity: Newton's Laws of Getting Stuff Done." James Clear. https://1ref.us/1ex (accessed May 11, 2020).

Clinton, Tim, and Max Davis. "Only God Can Fill the Void." DR. JAMES DOBSON'S family talk. https://1ref.us/1eg (accessed May 5, 2020).

"Complete Health Improvement Program." Lifestyle Medicine Institute (accessed July 9, 2020).

"*Confessions* (Augustine)." Wikipedia. https://1ref.us/1ef (accessed May 11, 2020).

Day, Lorraine. *You Can't Improve on God.* Thousand Palms, CA: Rockford Press, 1997.

"Diabetes: The rice you eat is worse than sugary drinks." The Straits Times. https://1ref.us/1fb (accessed May 11, 2020).

Fernandez, Alvaro, Elkhonon Goldberg, and Pascale Michelon. "Neuroplasticity: the potential for lifelong brain development." Sharp Brains. https://1ref.us/1fh (accessed April 15, 2020).

"Four crucial ways that sleep helps the body to heal." Chicago Tribune. https://1ref.us/1f2 (accessed July 9, 2020).

Gamow, G. *The Creation of the Universe.* New York, NY: Dover Publications, 1952.

"Giving thanks can make you happier." Harvard Health Publishing. https://1ref.us/1eq (accessed April 15, 2020), (emphasis added).

Hardinge, M. *A Philosophy of Health.* Loma Linda, CA: School of Health, Loma Linda University, 1980.

King, Barbara. "Humans are 'Meathooked' But Not Designed For Meat-Eating." National Public Radio. https://1ref.us/1f7 (accessed May 11, 2020).

Laskowski, Edward R. "How much should the average adult exercise every day?" Mayo Clinic. https://1ref.us/1ez (accessed May 11, 2020).

Levterov, Theodore. "A True Prophet …." Adventist. https://1ref.us/1fk (accessed May 7, 2020).

"Lifestyle Choices to Boost immunity." American College of Lifestyle Medicine. https://1ref.us/1f4 (accessed May 11, 2020).

"Live More," Lifestyle Medicine Institute, https://1ref.us/1f6 (accessed July 9, 2020).

Lowell, James Russel. Quotes.pub. https://1ref.us/1ew (accessed May 11, 2020).

McAndrew, Frank T. "Why high school stays with us forever." The Conversation. https://1ref.us/1er (accessed May 11, 2020).

Mineo, Liz. "Good genes are nice, but joy is better." Harvard Gazette. https://1ref.us/1es (accessed May 11, 2020).

Moore, Russell. "Does Jeremiah 29:11 Apply to You?" The Gospel Coalition. https://1ref.us/1eu (accessed May 11, 2020).

Morneau, Roger. *Incredible Answers to Prayer.* Hagerstown, MD: Review and Herald Publishing Association, 1990.

Nall, Rachel. "What Are the Benefits of Sunlight?" healthline. https://1ref.us/1ek (accessed May 11, 2020).

"*Pale Blue Dot.*" Wikipedia. https://1ref.us/1fi (accessed April 15, 2020).

Pascal, B. *Pensées.* New York, NY: Penguin Books, 1966.

Paulien, Gunther B. *The Divine Prescription and Science of Health and Healing.* New York, NY: TEACH Services, Inc, 1995.

Petre, Alina. "How to Follow a Raw Vegan Diet: Benefits and Risks." healthline. https://1ref.us/1f9 (accessed May 11, 2020).

"Physical Properties of Water." Physical Geography. https://1ref.us/1eo (accessed May 11, 2020).

Raymond, Joseph R. "Nutrition Sayings and Quotes." Wise Old Sayings. https://1ref.us/1f3 (accessed July 9, 2020).

Rodriguez, Ángel M. "The health-reform program contributes to manifest God's loving concern for humankind." Perspective Digest. https://1ref.us/1ee (accessed May 5, 2020).

Roser, Max, Esteban Ortiz-Ospina, and Hannah Ritchie. "Life Expectancy." Our World in Data. https://1ref.us/1fg (accessed April 15, 2020).

"Rule of threes (survival)." Wikipedia. https://1ref.us/1ej (accessed May 11, 2020).

Russell, Chris. "8 Keys to Knowing God's Will For Your Life." Bible Study Tools. https://1ref.us/1ev (accessed May 11, 2020).

Sagan, Carol. "A Pale Blue Dot." The Planetary Society. https://1ref.us/1fj (accessed April 15, 2020).

Sammis, John H. "Trust and Obey." Seventh-day Adventist Hymnal. Review and Herald Publishing Association, 1985.

Santhanam, Laura. "American life expectancy has dropped again. Here's why." PBS News Hour. https://1ref.us/1ff (accessed April 15, 2020).

Sarbadhikari, Suptendra N., and Asit K. Saha. "Moderate exercise and chronic stress produce counteractive effects on different areas of the brain by acting through various neurotransmitter receptor subtypes: A hypothesis." National Center for Biotechnology Information. https://1ref.us/1f1 (accessed May 11, 2020).

Saxe, J. *The poems of John Godfrey Saxe.* Boston, MA: Houghton, Mifflin and Company, 1881.

Silverthorn, Dee U. *Human Physiology: An Integrated Approach.* 4th ed. San Francisco, CA: Pearson Education, Inc, 2009.

Terranova, Jacob. "The Sunshine Supplement: Understanding Vitamin D and the Sun." THORNE. https://1ref.us/1el (accessed May 11, 2020).

"The 4 Components of a good exercise programme." health24. https://1ref.us/1ey (accessed May 11, 2020).

The GARDENS© integrated model of health promotion and education was formulated by Libni A. Cerdenio as the framework for the wholistic health teaching ministry of Wellness Plus Institute.

The Sound of Music. Directed and produced by Robert Wise, 20th Century Fox, 1965.

"The Water in You: Water and the Human Body." USGS. https://1ref.us/1em (accessed May 11, 2020).

Tuso, Philip, Mohamed Ismail, Benjamin Ha, and Carole Bartolotto, "Nutritional Update for Physicians: Plant-Based Diets." National Center for Biotechnology Information. https://1ref.us/1f5 (accessed May 11, 2020).

"Vegetarian Diets Associated With Lower Risk of Death." JAMA Network. https://1ref.us/1f8 (accessed May 11, 2020).

Wagner, Gina D. "Strength in Numbers: The Importance of Fitness Buddies." 2Unstoppable. https://1ref.us/1f0 (accessed May 11, 2020).

Walsh, Anthony. *Answering the New Atheists: How Science Points to God and to the Benefits of Christianity.* Wilmington, DE: Vernon Press, 2019.

"Water: Essential to your body." MAYO CLINIC HEALTH SYSTEM. https://1ref.us/1en (accessed May 11, 2020).

"What are clean and unclean foods?" Bible Study. https://1ref.us/1fa (accessed May 11, 2020).

"What does it mean that the wise man built his house upon a rock?" Got Questions, https://1ref.us/1fv (accessed November 5, 2020).

"WHEN IS THE BEST TIME TO EAT BREAKFAST, LUNCH, AND DINNER?" Forklift and Palate. https://1ref.us/1fc (accessed May 11, 2020).

White, Ellen G. *Christ's Object Lessons.* Mountain View, CA: Pacific Press Publishing Association, 1900.

White, Ellen G. *Christ Triumphant.* Hagerstown, MD: Review and Herald Publishing Association, 1999.

White, Ellen G. *Counsels on Diet and Foods.* Washington, DC: Review and Herald Publishing Association, 1938.

White, Ellen G. *Counsels on Health.* Mountain View, CA: Pacific Press Publishing Association, 1923.

White, Ellen G. *Education.* Mountain View, CA: Pacific Press Publishing Association, 1903.

White, Ellen G. *God's Amazing Grace.* Hagerstown, MD: Review and Herald Publishing Association, 1973.

White, Ellen G. *Healthful Living.* Battle Creek, MI: Medical Missionary Board, 1897.

White, Ellen G. *Mind, Character, and Personality*. Vol. 1. Hagerstown, MD: Review and Herald Publishing Association, 1977.

White, Ellen G. *Mind, Character, and Personality*, Vol. 2. Hagerstown, MD: Review and Herald Publishing Association, 1977.

White, Ellen G. *Prayer.* Nampa, ID: Pacific Press Publishing Association, 2002.

White, Ellen G. *Reflecting Christ.* Hagerstown, MD: Review and Herald Publishing Association, 2008.

White, Ellen G. *Sons and Daughters of God.* Hagerstown, MD: Review and Herald Publishing Association, 1983.

White, Ellen G. *Steps to Christ.* Mountain View, CA: Pacific Press Publishing Association, 1892.

White, Ellen G. "Steps to Jesus." EGW Writings. https://m.egwwritings. org/en/book/2017.508#527 (accessed June 23, 2020).

White, Ellen G. *The Ministry of Healing.* Mountain View, CA: Pacific Press Publishing Association, 1905.

Wong, J.B. *Christian Wholism: Theological and Ethical Implications in the Postmodern World.* Lanham, MD: University Press of America, 2002.

TEACH Services, Inc.
P U B L I S H I N G

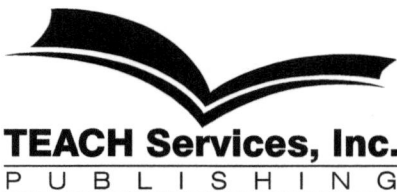

We invite you to view the complete
selection of titles we publish at:
www.TEACHServices.com

We encourage you to write us
with your thoughts about this,
or any other book we publish at:
info@TEACHServices.com

TEACH Services' titles may be purchased in
bulk quantities for educational, fund-raising,
business, or promotional use.
bulksales@TEACHServices.com

Finally, if you are interested in seeing
your own book in print, please contact us at:
publishing@TEACHServices.com
We are happy to review your manuscript at no charge.

www.ingramcontent.com/pod-product-compliance
Lightning Source LLC
Chambersburg PA
CBHW040136270326
41927CB00019B/3407